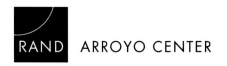

RAND ARROYO CENTER

T0131044

Core Competencies for Amputation Rehabilitation

Jason Michel Etchegaray, Heather Krull, Stephanie Brooks Holliday,
Lea Xenakis, Bernard D. Rostker, Nahom M. Beyene,
Sangeeta C. Ahluwalia, Tepring Piquado, Edward W. Chan,
Angela Clague

Prepared for the United States Army
Approved for public release; distribution unlimited

For more information on this publication, visit **www.rand.org/t/RR2898**

Library of Congress Cataloging-in-Publication Data is available for this publication.
ISBN: 978-1-9774-0223-3

Support RAND
Make a tax-deductible charitable contribution at
www.rand.org/giving/contribute

www.rand.org

Preface

This report documents research and analysis conducted as part of a project entitled *Core Competencies for Amputation Rehabilitation*, sponsored by the U.S. Army Medical Command. The purpose of this study was to identify which services are integral to optimal amputee care and to define and document core competencies for each of these services to guide clinical rehabilitative care for service members who experience deployment-related extremity amputation(s).

The Project Unique Identification Code (PUIC) for the project that produced this document is RAN167321.

This research was conducted within the RAND Arroyo Center's Personnel, Training, and Health Program. RAND Arroyo Center, part of the RAND Corporation, is a federally funded research and development center (FFRDC) sponsored by the United States Army.

RAND operates under a "Federal-Wide Assurance" (FWA00003425) and complies with the *Code of Federal Regulations for the Protection of Human Subjects Under United States Law* (45 CFR 46), also known as "the Common Rule," as well as with the implementation guidance set forth in Department of Defense (DOD) Instruction 3216.02. As applicable, this compliance includes reviews and approvals by RAND's Institutional Review Board (the Human Subjects Protection Committee) and by the U.S. Army. The views of sources utilized in this study are solely their own and do not represent the official policy or position of DOD or the U.S. government.

Contents

Figures

Tables

Summary

After the United States was attacked on 9/11, the Army Surgeon General recognized the need to prepare for the care and rehabilitation that would be required by those who experienced deployment-related amputation(s). The Army set to work quickly to establish a system that could handle their complex wounds; by late 2001, the Surgeon General approved the development of a "virtual" amputee system of care, and a panel of outside experts was developing a plan for how to treat these patients. In mid-2002, the Army Surgeon General approved Walter Reed Army Medical Center (WRAMC) as the Army's primary location to care for patients who experienced amputation. Brooke Army Medical Center became DOD's secondary site, and eventually, Naval Medical Center San Diego (NMCSD) became the third. By 2007, all three rehabilitation centers (Center for the Intrepid [CFI] in San Antonio, Texas, Comprehensive Combat and Complex Casualty Care [C5] in San Diego, California, and Advanced Amputee Training Center [AATC] in Washington, D.C., which later became Military Advanced Training Center [MATC] in Bethesda, Maryland) were fully operational. Since that time, DOD has provided state-of-the-science rehabilitation to over 2,000 service members who have experienced amputation(s).[1]

As measured by the number of service members who required care for new amputation(s) sustained in or after combat, 2011 was a peak year. As a consequence of lower deployment operational tempo (OPTEMPO), the number of new amputations has shrunk in each subsequent year, with 16 amputation patients in 2014 and even fewer since. In order to capture best practices and the knowledge, skills, abilities, and other (KSAO) that were developed by DOD and the providers who rehabilitated these patients, the Extremity Trauma and Amputation Center of Excellence (EACE) asked RAND Arroyo Center to identify the services that are integral to optimal amputation rehabilitation and to define and document the core competencies that are needed by health care providers who offer those services. This report contains the results of that effort.

---

[1] As of November 2018, the current number of active duty service members with major amputation was 2,147.

Methods and Findings

RAND Arroyo Center worked with the sponsor and stakeholders to identify an initial list of services perceived to be integral to optimal amputation rehabilitation. Then the team interviewed approximately 110 patients, family members, health care providers, and subject matter experts to learn about the behaviors observed in the providers who rehabilitate this patient population, areas at risk of skill atrophy when providers are not seeing enough of these patients, and best practices among the care team and more generally within the military treatment facilities where amputation rehabilitation occurs. The research team transcribed and coded the interviews, which, together with existing competency frameworks and/or practice standards and information from the *Care of the Combat Amputee* (Lenhart, Pasquina, and Cooper, 2009), resulted in an initial list of competencies that are needed by providers in nine areas of rehabilitation: behavioral health, case management, diet/nutrition, occupational therapy, orthopaedic surgery, physical therapy (PT), physical medicine and rehabilitation, prosthetics and orthotics, and biomedical engineering. For each service, the research team also identified exemplar behaviors that, when observed, demonstrate that the provider possesses that competency. These initial competencies and behaviors were presented in the form of a technical expert survey (TES) in two waves to providers in each service area. Upon completion of the TES, the research team finalized the core competencies that are common to these nine areas of rehabilitation, as shown in Figure S.1. For each service area, there is a set of behaviors that accompanies each competency.

Recommendations

With a set of core competencies and behaviors for nine services necessary for amputation rehabilitation, we offer five recommendations on how to adopt and implement these competencies in the military health setting.

Our first recommendation is that **core competencies need to be formally accepted by those leading and working in military health care settings**. That requires Military Health System (MHS) leadership to become champions of these competencies and for leaders, administrators, and health care providers to buy into the importance of the competency framework and the behaviors that demonstrate that those providing rehabilitative services possess the competencies.

Next, we recommend that, **once accepted, those in military health care settings must decide how to use competencies**. We developed a competency model, consisting of competencies and related behaviors, that provides an organizing framework for behaviors that one needs to perform for a given job. Therefore, the findings of this study may be applied in several ways, including but not limited to hiring decisions, performance appraisal, and identifying training needs. As an example, in

Figure S.1
RAND Arroyo Center Competencies for Deployment-Related Amputation Rehabilitation

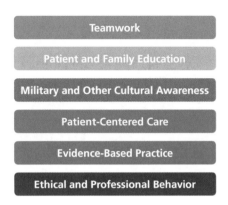

the early 2000s, Army Medical Command (MEDCOM) developed and posted competency assessments/tools for several health care provider positions, which are used to document six types of information about such matters as job descriptions and evidence of competency assessment, professional education, military training and other achievements, information about licensure and certification, and professional experience. These assessments are called *six-sided folders*. Given that MEDCOM has already developed the format and recommended way that the six-sided folders should be used, one way to incorporate competencies we identified into a performance appraisal process is to integrate these competencies into the existing framework.

Third, **MHS leadership should adopt a proficiency framework for assessing individual and system-wide competencies.** One such example is the National Academies of Sciences (NAS), Engineering, and Medicine's Five Levels of Clinical Competence Framework. The five levels are novice, advanced beginner, competent, proficient, and expert. This framework has at least two valuable functions as DOD begins to adopt and implement the core competencies developed in this study: It (1) establishes a desired distribution of proficiency that is needed to provide optimal rehabilitative services to patients with amputation and (2) conducts a baseline assessment of current staff. The desired skill level mix likely depends upon patient volume and patient need, both today and as projected into the future (in the event of future conflicts, for instance). Upon completion of the baseline assessment, if the current mix of clinical skill levels falls below or is otherwise misaligned with the desired distribution, MHS, EACE, and the Defense Health Agency (DHA) will be able to implement a plan for how to close the gap.

Our fourth recommendation is that **metrics and assessment time frames associated with competencies must be validated for military health care settings.** Once a baseline has been established for the current skill mix among providers who rehabilitate patients with amputation, individual providers and the overall mix of clinical competence should be assessed regularly. Assessment can occur in a number of ways, including (1) providers sharing examples of ways they demonstrate the behaviors in practice, (2) providers demonstrating the behaviors in simulation exercises, (3) peers sharing examples about providers demonstrating these competencies, and (4) patients providing input about the quality/quantity of these behaviors. The type of assessment conducted will vary by provider type or service, competency, and behavior. Some literature in this area recommends that "all staff should be assessed prior to employment, during the orientation period, and at least annually thereafter" (Kak, Burkhalter, and Cooper, 2001, p. 5).

Finally, **once optimal skill mix has been identified, competency gaps and mitigation strategies need to be developed**. The types of training needed to close the gap between a provider's current competency level and the desired level will depend upon the provider's specialty and his or her current clinical competence level, but may range from online courses, conference attendance, review of clinical practice guidelines and other resources, or rotations to civilian trauma centers or high-volume military treatment facilities.

The competencies developed in this study apply to a broad range of services and individual providers, each with its own set of documented behaviors that demonstrate mastery of a competency, and they provide a framework for assessing DOD's current mix of skills among providers who rehabilitate patients with amputation(s) related to combat experience. Where gaps exist between current and desired levels of clinical competency, a variety of training opportunities already exist or could be developed to ensure that service members wounded in future conflicts will experience the same or better state-of-the-art rehabilitative services than veterans of Operation Enduring Freedom (OEF) and Operation Iraqi Freedom (OIF) received.

Acknowledgments

This research was sponsored by Mr. John Shero, Extremity Trauma and Amputation Center of Excellence (EACE). His direction and feedback throughout the study helped shape it along the way. Mr. James Mundy, EACE, provided support as the study began and over the course of the entire project. Dr. Andrea Crunkhorn, EACE, served as the action officer and provided guidance every step of the way, for which the study team is tremendously grateful.

At each of the DOD facilities we visited, individuals went out of their way to assist with our visit and help identify potential interviewees. Mr. Stuart Campbell and Dr. Chris Dearth, EACE, hosted us on multiple trips to CFI and assisted us with understanding the center's mission as well as introducing us to providers. Although we did not interview health care providers from the Department of Veterans Affairs (VA), three experts who were partially or completely affiliated with the VA's Amputation System of Care—Dr. Billie J. Randolph, Dr. Joseph Miller, and Dr. Joseph Webster— met with us to provide information about the VA's amputation patient population and how VA manages their care, which was valuable for our research about how DOD can maintain and improve its care to this patient population.

The analysis would not have been possible without input from the many patients, health care providers, and subject matter experts throughout DOD and the civilian sector. We are grateful to all of the individuals who participated in one-on-one interviews and/or completed the TESs that helped us refine and gather initial evidence for the validity of competencies for amputation rehabilitation. In addition, we visited four civilian rehabilitation centers—Spaulding Rehabilitation Hospital, Shirley Ryan AbilityLab, The Institute for Rehabilitation and Research (TIRR) Memorial Hermann, and Shepherd Center—to learn about their best practices in amputation rehabilitation. Each site offered us one to two days to tour the facilities and to interview leadership and individual providers. We are grateful for the time and insights into how care is delivered in their impressive facilities.

Finally, several RAND researchers made important contributions to this study. Ritika Chaturvedi, Melinda Moore, Rajeev Ramchand, Alfonso Rivera, and Ellen Tunstall collected data for it, either through published literature or by conducting interviews. Prior to administering the TES, the study team tested the protocol with a group of RAND behavioral health researchers. We are grateful to Lynsay Ayer, Michael Dunbar, Nicole Eberhart, Coreen Farris, Karen Osilla, and Christine Vaughan for their input. Finally, Jayne Gordon's assistance in scheduling interviews and site visits was extremely helpful.

Carra Sims of RAND and Seth Messinger of the University of Washington reviewed a draft of this report, and their feedback helped to improve it tremendously.

Abbreviations

AVF	all-volunteer force
AW2	Army Wounded Warrior Program
BAMC	Brooke Army Medical Center
BRAC	Base Realignment and Closure
C5	Comprehensive Combat and Complex Casualty Care
CAF	competency assessment file
CanMEDS	Canadian Medical Education Directives for Specialists
CAREN	Computer-Assisted Rehab Environment
CBD	Competence by Design
CFI	Center for the Intrepid
COAD	continuance on active duty
DARPA	Defense Advanced Research Projects Agency
DHA	Defense Health Agency
DHB	Defense Health Board
DOD	Department of Defense
DS3	Disabled Soldier Support System
EACE	Extremity Trauma and Amputation Center of Excellence
FTE	full-time equivalent
FY	fiscal year
ICF	International Classification of Functioning, Disability, and Health
IED	improvised explosive device
IOM	Institute of Medicine
KSAO	knowledge, skills, abilities, and other
MATC	Military Advanced Training Center
MEB	medical evaluation board
MEDCOM	Medical Command
MHS	Military Health System
MTF	Military Treatment Facility
NAS	National Academies of Sciences
NIH	National Institutes of Health

NMCSD	Naval Medical Center San Diego
OEF	Operation Enduring Freedom
OIF	Operation Iraqi Freedom
OND	Operation New Dawn
OTSG	Office of the Surgeon General
PEB	physical evaluation board
PM&R	physical medicine and rehabilitation
POC	point of contact
PT	physical therapy, physical therapist
PTSD	posttraumatic stress disorder
SAH	single axis hydraulic
TBI	traumatic brain injury
TES	technical expert survey
TIRR	The Institute for Rehabilitation and Research Memorial Hermann
USAAPCP	United States Army Amputee Patient Care Program
VA	Department of Veterans Affairs
WHS	Washington Headquarters Service
WRAMC	Walter Reed Army Medical Center
WRNMMC	Walter Reed National Military Medical Center

CHAPTER ONE

Introduction

The way the nation cares for its war casualties today, both during their service and as veterans, is the result of progress along a well-established path that extends back to the eighteenth century and has seen improvements in both the quality of medical care and the availability of services provided for the rehabilitation of the combat amputee. Medical capabilities and experience treating the war wounded peak during periods of intense combat and tend to erode during interwar periods. The current conflicts in Iraq and Afghanistan have resulted in the largest number of U.S. casualties since the war in Vietnam. In the process, the clinical characteristics and health needs of the current war wounded population have been changing, with death rates and amputations at an all-time low. In past conflicts, the most serious battle injuries were typically wounds resulting from gun and artillery fire. Today's improvised explosive devices (IEDs), planted along roadsides, are the scourge of the battlefield. They often result in burns, traumatic brain injuries (TBIs), or limb loss (or some combination of the three).[1] Changes in battlefield medical technologies have profoundly changed the treatment of wounded service members. Rapid evacuation of the seriously wounded from the battlefield to the continental United States in a matter of days rather than weeks or months means that initial treatment and early rehabilitative services can now take place at state-of-the-art medical centers at home, rather than overseas.

Between 2001 and 2014, 1,640 service members experienced major limb amputations as part of conflicts in Afghanistan, Iraq, and Syria. The peak years, as measured by new deployment-related amputations, were 2007 (213 service members) and 2011 (260 service members), with the number of major limb amputations steadily declining since 2011. These deployment-related amputations are different from amputations resulting from other types of injuries or illnesses, as noted by

---

[1] The IEDs used in Iraq were often made out of artillery shells. They were used like land mines and produced similar casualties. At the end of World War II, the increased use of land mines by the retreating Germans resulted in a significant increase of wounds to the lower extremities. In 1943, 15 percent of all amputations were attributed to land mines; by the last year of the war (1944–1945), the rate more than doubled to 34 percent (Hampton, 1957).

Charles Scoville, then-chief of the Walter Reed Army Medical Center (WRAMC)–
Amputee Care Center:

> The wounding patterns resulting from military conflict are very different from
> civilian injuries and have a great impact on the management of the associated
> amputations. The high kinetic energy delivered by modern munitions results in
> extensive soft tissue zones of injury, causing wounds that are subject to more com-
> plications, and may take longer to heal. These munitions focus their destructive
> forces on the extremity creating a particularly complex wound where fragments of
> the munitions and other debris are driven into the affected limb. The blast wave
> peels away the clothing or boot and soft tissues, crushing bone and then stripping
> it. Left behind is exposed bone with a flap of skin and other soft tissue. Debris has
> been driven between fascial planes along the path of least resistance. This is not
> just a simple amputation and has no real counterpart in civilian trauma. War inju-
> ries often have much more soft tissue damage than is initially apparent. Failure to
> investigate these fascial planes or premature closure of these wounds will inevitably
> lead to sepsis and the need to re-amputate at a higher, less functional level. This
> severe damage to the soft tissue envelope may require higher amputation levels to
> prevent infection and allow for bone coverage. The munitions used in a military
> conflict are also capable of causing extensive injury to multiple extremities, result-
> ing in the amputation of more than one limb.
>
> Wounds related to war surgery are initially left open because of the high risk of
> infection. A staged approach to amputation surgery is necessary to obtain wound
> closure and a residual limb that can provide the best function. Because of the
> severe nature of war wounds, reconstructive procedures are often done later, even
> months after injury. If extensive soft tissue or bone procedures are done before the
> soft tissue envelope has recovered and stabilized, there is a higher risk of infection,
> failure and a higher level of amputation. Blast injuries also may have associated
> mild-moderate traumatic brain injuries (TBI) that are concomitant with amputa-
> tions. TBIs seem to result from initial blast, concussive effects within the skull,
> and injury from the brain/skull complex hitting the ground. We perform TBI test-
> ing to detect cognitive and other deficits, which can affect each amputee's short-
> and long-term rehab course. (Scoville, 2003g, p. 1)

The large number of complex injuries being sustained by service members and a
change in the Army's strategy for caring for such patients resulted in the development
in 2001 of "virtual" amputation-specific centers to provide consistent treatment to
patients anchored around the WRAMC as the initial center of care, with Brooke Army
Medical Center (BAMC) being approved as another center of care in 2002. The effort
of the Department of Defense (DOD) to develop these centers allowed for patients
to receive comprehensive treatment from a team of health care providers focused on
amputation rehabilitation. Patient volume from combat has decreased since 2011, and
as with previous interwar periods, provider skills and proficiency to treat and rehabili-

Figure 1.1
Individuals with Major Limb Amputations due to Battle Injuries in Operation Iraqi Freedom, Operation New Dawn, Operation Inherent Resolve, Operation Enduring Freedom, and Operation Freedom's Sentinel, October 7, 2001–June 1, 2015

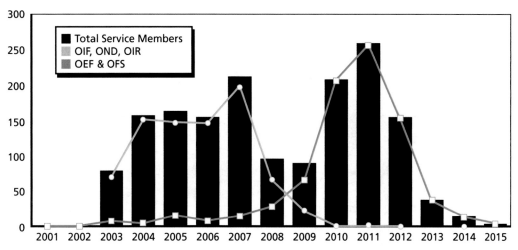

SOURCE: Fischer, 2015.
NOTES: OIF = Operation Iraqi Freedom, OND = Operation New Dawn, OIR = Operation Inherent Resolve, OEF = Operation Enduring Freedom, and OFS = Operation Freedom's Sentinel.

tate these patients are likely to atrophy in the absence of efforts to mitigate skill erosion. To prepare for future conflict and increased patient volume, the military medical community must identify ways to maintain and improve skills during this period of low-patient volume.

To capture the lessons learned from caring for this patient population over the last 17 years and prevent atrophy of knowledge, skills, abilities, and other (KSAO) due to small numbers of patients currently experiencing deployment-related limb loss, the U.S. Army Medical Command and the joint DOD–Department of Veterans Affairs (VA) Extremity Trauma and Amputation Center of Excellence (EACE) asked RAND Arroyo Center to develop and document core competencies needed for services DOD provides for amputation rehabilitation.

This research supports many ongoing efforts. At the time it was initiated, The Military Health System's (MHS) *Strategic Plan* (The Military Health System, 2014) was focused on improved readiness, better health, better care, and lower cost. This research, which documents the core competencies that providers who rehabilitate patients with deployment-related amputation must have, supports at least three MHS *Strategic Plan* initiatives: (1) maintain a ready medical force, (2) improve clinical outcomes and consistent patient experience, and (3) improve condition-based quality care. In addition, the Defense Health Board (DHB) reviewed amputee care and developed findings and recommendations about future needs in such care, which are documented in its 2015 report titled *Sustainment and Advancement of Amputee Care*. One of the DHB's findings was that while DOD provides excellent care to service members experiencing amputations, it must understand the core competencies needed for optimal rehabilitation services. The DHB's recommendation was that

> DOD must ensure sustainment of the highest quality delivery of health care and health research in spite of post-conflict resource limitations. Core competencies in optimal amputee care must be defined, periodically updated, tracked, and regularly reported to the leadership of the Military Health System. (DHB, 2015, p. 7)

Our study addresses this recommendation by identifying and documenting core competencies needed by health care providers who rehabilitate service members with amputations.

An inherent assumption in this research is that the care that was delivered to this patient population and the skills acquired by providers while caring for them represent what competencies should be captured and what DOD aims to repeat (and improve upon) in future conflicts. In other words, we assume that by establishing an amputee system of care, anchored initially at WRAMC and expanded to BAMC and eventually the Naval Medical Center San Diego (NMCSD), DOD achieved its goal of providing the highest quality care. Although we treat this as an assumption, based on the genesis of this research to document competencies for purpose of sustaining the highest quality delivery of health care, we acknowledge that it is something that ought to be evaluated.

One way to assess the care that DOD provided to patients with deployment-related amputations is to examine patient outcomes, such as functional restoration, quality of life, and return to duty. Appendix B provides an overview of some of this literature, but we will also highlight it here. It is important to note that the studies mentioned here are not specifically about patient outcomes associated with care provided by DOD; rather, they concern outcomes among veterans of Operation Enduring Freedom (OEF) and Operation Iraqi Freedom (OIF).

A national survey of Vietnam War, OEF, and OIF amputees entitled "Survey for Prosthetic Use" (Department of Veterans Affairs, Office of Rehabilitation Research and Development undated) has been used by several researchers to study how service members do and do not use their prosthetic devices. Gailey et al. (2010) found that three factors—increasing numbers of specialty prosthetic devices in current use, higher overall quality of life, and higher number of total devices ever received—were associated with higher functional ability among OEF and OIF survey respondents with lower limb loss. DOD's amputation rehabilitation program generously fits patients with a variety of prosthetics, as needed by the service member or veteran, and these findings suggest that this policy results in improved functioning. Use of prosthetic devices varied depending upon whether the amputation was upper or lower limb. Gailey et al. (2010) found that 4 percent of lower limb OEF/OIF veterans abandoned their prosthetic, compared to 22 percent among those with upper limb amputation(s) (McFarland et al., 2010). Epstein, Heinemann, and McFarland (2010) examined quality of life among OEF/OIF veterans and found that nearly 50 percent of male respondents reported excellent or very good quality of life. Needing assistance with activities of daily living was correlated with worse overall quality of life. Finally, multiple studies have reported return to duty rates among OEF/OIF veterans, including that of Stinner et al. (2010), who found an overall rate of 16.5 percent among soldiers, with transtibial amputees representing one of the largest shares of the sample who also have one of the highest rates of return to duty (22 percent). Hurley et al. (2015) found that 13 percent of OIF/OEF/Operation New Dawn (OND) veterans who were evaluated for disability were found fit for duty, either remaining in their primary occupation or continuing on active duty in a less physically demanding role. There are also more qualitatively oriented outcomes that can be examined. For example, Messinger (2009) used a case study approach to examine reasons why prosthetic devices are accepted by some patients and rejected by others, with key findings indicating that the structure of the rehabilitation program (i.e., extent to which it is focused on improving physical functioning) and patient perceptions of autonomy affect whether devices are used by patients.

We return to the issue of measuring patient outcomes at the conclusion of this report.

Study Approach

Care for patients who experience a deployment-related amputation begins in theater at the point of injury. In some cases, the limb is lost when the injury occurs, but in others, the amputation occurs later in the care process, including once the service member is medically evacuated out of theater or after a period of recovery with a salvaged limb. Because of the varied paths that these patients take to recovery and rehabilitation, we elected, with input from EACE leadership, to limit the study to rehabilitation that occurs postoperatively through reintegration into regular activities such as work. Care that is delivered preoperatively and the maintenance that occurs after reintegration were outside the scope of research. Figure 1.2 displays and describes the seven phases of care published by the Amputee Coalition of America (Highsmith and Kahle, 2008) and indicates the ones included in our analysis. Our study focused on many of the stages of rehabilitation that service members experience; we use the term *care* to denote the services provided to patients during such rehabilitation.

For the purposes of this study, rather than thinking about care provided by an individual provider or type of provider, we considered *services*. For instance, an occupational therapist or certified occupational therapy assistant can provide occupa-

Figure 1.2
Amputee Coalition Phases of Care

Preoperative phase (out of scope)	Postoperative phase	Preprosthetic phase	Preparatory prosthetic training phase	Definitive prosthetic training phase	Reintegration phase	Maintenance (out of scope)
	• "The emphasis here is balancing recovery from the traumatic or surgical amputation(s) by protecting healing and beginning to shape the residual limb(s) while encouraging activity and mobility as soon as possible." • May include serial surgical washouts, extended care for infection, treatment to concomitant injuries, and multiple amputations in different phases at any one point in time.	• "By now, general activity and possibly mobility without a prosthesis hopefully is progressing well. This phase focuses largely on aerobic conditioning, strengthening the entire body, flexibility and final shaping of the residual limb(s) for eventual fitting of the preparatory prosthesis(es)." • This phase may be achieved for one limb while other limb trauma or amputation remains in an earlier phase. This is prevalent with intractable infections.	• "Many basic prosthetic skills must be learned before and during early weight-bearing activities in the prosthesis(es)." • This phase is lengthened for multiple-limb amputees.	• "As the individual progresses into these later phases, the therapy becomes more individually tailored given individual circumstances, components and, above all, goals." • This is the most intensive rehabilitation phase for DOD amputees, focusing on individualized treatment plans to optimize individual functional outcomes.	• "In this phase, the individual is preparing to return to specific activities such as work or recreation or may need help in training for new activities."	

SOURCE: Highsmith and Kahle, 2008, pp. 30–34.

tional therapy services. Similarly, a psychologist or psychiatrist could provide behavioral health services. Data collected during this study were combined and analyzed at the service level.

Definition of Competency

We begin by defining competencies to orient the reader to this construct and a related process used to understand competencies—competency modeling. Competencies are "nested" constructs that are unique, have multiple interrelated underlying behaviors, and are needed for successful job execution (Schippmann et al., 2000; Society for Human Resource Management, 2012). Competencies serve multiple roles, including (1) reflecting KSAOs important to a specific job and (2) allowing one to determine what behaviors to measure as indicative of the competency of interest. As a generic example of the nested nature of the relationship between competencies, KSAOs, and behaviors, a *competency* for physicians might be clinical proficiency. *Knowledge* of human anatomy is needed for a physician to have clinical proficiency, and a *behavior* that the physician demonstrates to show this might be treating an upper limb wound. Our conceptualization of a competency is consistent with DOD's Competency Management Framework, given that we focused on "observable, measurable pattern[s] of knowledge, skills, and abilities" that "include behaviors associated with job performance" (U.S. Department of Defense, 2016, p. 15).

Given EACE's interest in identifying and documenting competencies, we used a competency modeling approach, which is one way that psychologists and human resource professionals understand what one needs to do to be successful on a job. For this project, we identified *core* competencies across services provided during rehabilitation, which means that we were interested in competencies that were common to all (i.e., across) services provided during amputation rehabilitation.[2] One advantage of this approach is that we were able to look for commonalities across services via competencies while still maintaining uniqueness within type of service for each competency by identifying observable measures and/or behaviors reflecting specific KSAOs relevant to certain services. Identifying competencies is an initial step in helping organizations know what they should focus on when deciding how to train, assess, and develop personnel (Marrelli, Tondora, and Hoge, 2005). There are two important caveats to our methodology. First, we conducted interviews with individual health care providers responsible for providing amputation rehabilitation to this particular patient population whose injuries are complex (as described above) and who generally seek to return

---

[2]   Conceptually, this is consistent with DOD's Competency Management Framework, which specifies that core competencies "apply across DOD regardless of DOD Component or occupation" (DOD, 2016, p. 14). In the case of DOD Instruction 1400.25 (DOD, 2016), core competencies would extend beyond amputation rehabilitation, but that is not our intent in this study. Core competencies in the context of this research means that they apply to all of the providers included in our analysis while they rehabilitate patients with deployment-related amputation(s).

to a high level of fitness. Here, the time span between the height of war and date when we received approval to collect data meant that many providers who provided rehabilitation during the most recent wars were difficult to contact for various reasons (i.e., retired, left the military, and so on) and that those whom we did interview needed to rely on memory about what they did to provide high-quality rehabilitation. Second, competency modeling typically includes distinguishing good performance from bad or levels of competence within each competency. In this study, we did not make an explicit link between competencies and performance or skill level. The objective of this research was to document competencies and associated exemplar behaviors, and our recommendations at the end of this report address how DOD should link competencies and behaviors to performance.

Scope of the Study

A limiting factor in conducting competency modeling, which involves interviewing individuals in the disciplines for which competencies are being developed, analyzing the findings of those interviews and developing competencies from them, and validating those competencies with experts (through a technical expert survey [TES] in our case),[3] was the number and types of individuals in each discipline we were able to interview and the number who validated the competencies. Given Washington Headquarters Services (WHS) guidance in their approval process,[4] we focused on conducting at least five interviews for each service for which we developed competencies.[5] In the end, we developed competencies for the following rehabilitation services:

---

[3]   DOD (2016) describes DOD's Competency Management Advisory Group as being made up of subject matter experts from the Office of the Secretary of Defense (OSD), DOD component, and others, who support the implementation and sustainment of enterprise competencies. The approach used in this research is therefore consistent with DOD's civilian personnel management system.

[4]   We acquired several administrative approvals to conduct this research, including from primary and secondary institutional review boards, a Report Control Symbol from Washington Headquarters Services (WHS), and Paperwork Reduction Act through the Office and Management and Budget. In particular, WHS recommended a minimum sample size of five for "analysis/presentation of results." Where the total number of providers currently working at the three advanced rehabilitation centers was much larger than five, we interviewed more than five to obtain a more representative sample of responses.

[5]   Chapter Three provides additional information on the number of providers in each service category assigned to the three military treatment centers where most amputation rehabilitation takes place (Military Advanced Training Center [MATC], Center for the Intrepid [CFI], and Comprehensive Combat and Complex Casualty Care [C5]). As of May 2018, the size of these populations ranged from 0.5 full-time equivalent diet and nutrition providers to 17.25 individuals providing prosthetic and orthotic services. Our initial list consisted of orthopaedic surgery, physical medicine and rehabilitation, occupational therapy, physical therapy, prosthetics, case management, rehabilitation nurse specialist, psychological health (all disciplines), complex wound care team and dermatology, pain management, and peer visitor training. The final list excludes rehabilitation nurse specialist, complex wound care and dermatology, and peer visitor training due to too few potential participants available to be interviewed. In some case (i.e., nurses), we still obtained information about some specific tasks they perform related to rehabilitation (i.e., wound care) because these tasks were also performed by others.

- behavioral health (e.g., psychiatrists, psychologists)
- case management
- diet/nutrition
- occupational therapy
- orthopaedic surgery
- physical therapy
- physical medicine and rehabilitation
- prosthetics and orthotics
- biomedical engineering.

We now provide an overview of how the current literature defines competencies for the services we analyzed in this study.

Literature on Competencies Related to Amputation Rehabilitation

We reviewed the academic and gray literature[6] for competencies and associated behaviors for the rehabilitation services that we analyzed in this research.[7] We conducted this review to understand (1) what providers deemed valuable to amputation rehabilitation, (2) previous identification of competencies and behaviors for these providers, and (3) existing competency models from professional/association groups for these providers. This review and our identification of gaps also helped inform the development of interview guides, which we describe in Chapter Three.

First, there is a dearth of *peer-reviewed* literature on provider competencies and associated behaviors with respect to amputation rehabilitation. The majority of literature on competencies and underlying behaviors focuses on the types of providers who are part of an amputation rehabilitation team and not tailored specifically to caring for this patient population, which resulted in these authors discussing KSAOs (as opposed to competencies and behaviors) for the professions from a general, clinical perspective, rather than in terms of amputation rehabilitation specifically. Similarly, competencies for providers who treat trauma victims or rehabilitate those with disabilities are also largely absent from the literature. The absence of documented competencies for pro-

---

[6] Gray literature is that produced by organizations outside of the traditional commercial or academic publishing and distribution channels, and may include materials such as reports, theses, conference proceedings, working papers, government documents, white papers, and evaluations.

[7] This review was not limited to military research only and instead included behaviors documented for providers on the Occupational Information Network (O*NET), educational requirements for different provider types according to accrediting boards, and existing competency models. For the academic/gray search, we searched for three main constructs: (1) amputations, (2) provider types, and (3) knowledge, skills, abilities, and competencies. The primary academic database examined was PubMed, which is the National Library of Medicine's database of medical literature, and gray literature was examined via the Grey Literature Report. We also reviewed sources recommended to us by those we interviewed for this project (described below), such as the seminal book titled *Care of the Combat Amputee* (Lenhart, Pasquina, and Cooper, 2009).

viders who work with vulnerable patient populations, such as those who have experienced traumatic amputation, represents a major deficit in the literature. There is one non–peer reviewed publication, *Care of the Combat Amputee* (Lenhart, Pasquina, and Cooper, 2009), which details specific behaviors and KSAOs that we incorporated into our work.

Second, peer-reviewed literature seems to be primarily focused on providing information to patients who experienced amputations. For example, Australia has developed a roadmap of what patients should expect during the journey from surgery to reintegration based on a holistic Lifetime Support Scheme.[8] The Amputee Coalition of America provides resources and education to help patients understand amputations and related topics. The peer-reviewed literature also focuses on outcomes for those who experienced amputations, and while it is important, it is unrelated to our endeavor to identify and document core competencies.

We also examined U.S.-focused competency models to understand alternative ways that competencies are identified for providers and found two main types: (1) Institute of Medicine (IOM) and (2) provider-specific accrediting boards and/or graduate medical education programs. The IOM proposed a unifying competency framework that would apply to all health care providers and included five competencies: (1) providing patient-centered care, (2) working in interdisciplinary teams, (3) employing evidence-based practice, (4) applying quality improvement, and (5) utilizing informatics. Table 1.1 contains the competencies identified for different types of providers according to their boards/graduate programs.

As Table 1.1 shows, substantial variability exists in the competencies for the types of providers included in this research, yet a number of themes emerge. First, several include an element of teamwork or collaboration, including physicians (interpersonal and communication skills), prosthetists and orthotists (collaboration), case managers (facilitation, coordination, and collaboration), and rehabilitation psychologists (interpersonal interactions). Physicians and prosthetists/orthotists include practice-based and evidence-based care, respectively. Prosthetist and orthotist standards include competencies related to the patient and/or family member: patient-centered care and patient expectations. Both prosthetists/orthotists and physical therapists (PTs) are expected to educate (sharing knowledge for prosthetists/orthotists and education for PTs). Finally, physicians are unique in highlighting the importance of cultural competence.

Finally, several competency frameworks have been proposed internationally.

- The World Health Organization uses the International Classification of Functioning, Disability, and Health (ICF) to determine patient functioning and can

---

[8]   Government of South Australia, undated.

Table 1.1
Competency Frameworks from Accrediting Boards and Graduate Medical Education Programs

Provider Type	Competencies	Source
Physicians (Orthopaedic Surgeons, Physical Medicine and Rehabilitation, and Psychiatrists)	1. Patient Care and Procedural Skills 2. Medical Knowledge 3. Interpersonal and Communication Skills 4. Cultural Competence 5. Professionalism 6. Practice-Based Learning and Improvement 7. Systems-Based Practice	Accreditation Council for Graduate Medical Education, 2015
Prosthetists and Orthotists	1. Patient-Centered Care 2. Safety 3. Human Dignity 4. Integrative Practice 5. Collaboration 6. Evidence-Based Practice 7. Treatment Plan 8. Patient Expectations 9. Sharing Knowledge 10. Research Documentation 11. Clinical/Technical Procedures	National Commission on Orthotic and Prosthetic Education, 2010
Physical Therapists	1. Accountability 2. Professional Behavior 3. Professional Development 4. Examination, Evaluation, and Diagnosis 5. Plan of Care 6. Implementation 7. Education 8. Discharge	Federation of State Boards of Physical Therapy, 2006
Occupational Therapists	1. Professional Standing and Responsibility 2. Screening, Evaluation, and Re-Evaluation 3. Intervention 4. Outcomes	American Occupational Therapy Association, 2013
Biomedical Engineers	1. Professional Practice 2. Reliability, Safety, and Failure Analysis 3. Design 4. Engineering Tools 5. Engineering Knowledge 6. Biological Systems 7. Materials 8. Advanced Thermodynamics and Fluids 9. Power and Energy Systems 10. Control Theory and Systems	University of Victoria, undated

Table 1.1—Continued

Provider Type		Competencies	Source
Case Managers	1.	Client Selection Process for Case Management	Case Management Society of America, 2016
	2.	Client Assessment	
	3.	Problem/Opportunity Identification	
	4.	Planning	
	5.	Monitoring	
	6.	Facilitation, Coordination, and Collaboration	
	7.	Outcomes	
	8.	Termination of Case Management Services	
	9.	Qualifications for Case Managers	
	10.	Legal	
	11.	Confidentiality and Client Privacy	
Rehabilitation Psychologists	1.	Interpersonal Interactions	Stiers et al., 2015
	2.	Individual and Cultural Diversity	
	3.	Ethical and Legal Foundations	
	4.	Professional Identification	
	5.	Scientific Base and Knowledge	
	6.	Assessment	
	7.	Intervention	
	8.	Consultation	
	9.	Consumer Protection	

be helpful for medical students to begin to understand the association between disease and patient functioning.

- In the Netherlands, the Canadian Medical Education Directives for Specialists (CanMEDS) competency framework is used. Accordingly, Dutch physicians need to be skilled in seven different roles; the first, medical expert, incorporates the remaining six: professional, communicator, manager, health advocate, collaborator, and scholar.
- The General Assembly of the Dutch Society for Physical Medicine and Rehabilitation (PM&R) (Geertzen, Rommers, and Dekker, 2011) combined the ICF and CanMEDS models to delineate three levels of competencies (below, meet, exceed) and five levels of knowledge (has knowledge, needs direct supervision, needs global supervision, does not need supervision, supervises/teaches others).
- The Royal College of Physicians and Surgeons of Canada proposed the Competence by Design (CBD) Competence Continuum depicted in Figure 1.3. The foundational and core competencies are initially learned by students during the "Foundations of Discipline" and "Core of Discipline" stages, respectively, and then mastered during subsequent stages.

The lack of KSAOs, competencies, and behaviors identified specifically for amputation rehabilitation from the peer-reviewed literature highlights the importance of this

Figure 1.3
Competence by Design Competence Continuum

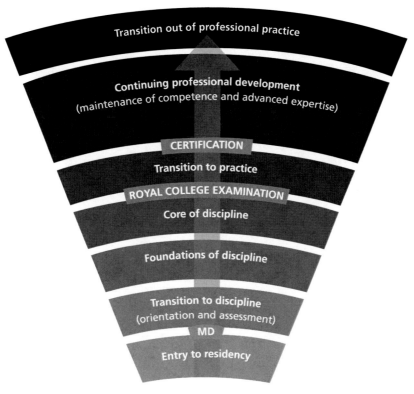

SOURCE: Royal College of Physicians and Surgeons of Canada, undated.
NOTE: Milestones at each stage describe terminal competencies.

current research. With a shrinking (new) patient population within DOD, it is critical that this information be documented before too much institutional knowledge is lost with natural staff turnover; the remainder of this report summarizes the findings of that effort.

Organization of the Report

We provide a brief history in Chapter Two of how DOD's care for patients with amputation has evolved since September 11, 2001. Chapter Three documents our competency modeling approach and results. Chapter 4 describes lessons learned from site visits to civilian rehabilitation centers. Chapter Five concludes with a range of options for how DOD can maintain and grow the capabilities it has developed in amputation care during the conflicts in Afghanistan, Iraq, and Syria.

CHAPTER TWO

Amputation Rehabilitation Since September 11, 2001

In this chapter, we provide an overview of the evolution of DOD's provision of rehabilitation for service members with amputations since 9/11,[1] including changes in DOD's approach to rehabilitation and the development of three advanced rehabilitation centers where much of the rehabilitation takes place. The new centers reflect the shift in how the Army has come to view service members who have experienced amputation(s): Whereas they were previously discharged from service, now they are treated as wounded warriors often fit to continue their military service.

Developing a System of Excellence in Amputation Rehabilitation

When the United States was attacked on September 11, 2001, the Army, and the entire DOD were unprepared to provide rehabilitation services to those who would soon experience combat-related amputations because of the uniqueness and complexity of their wounds (as described in Chapter One). After September 11, with the prospect of further conflict in the Middle East and in the anticipation of a new influx of amputees, the Army Surgeon General, Lieutenant General James Peake asked "for an estimate on the number of amputee patients that could be expected from a war in Afghanistan" (Scoville, 2007a) and a plan for how they should be handled. The staff of the Office of the Surgeon General (OTSG) understood the challenges as they prepared their recommendations for the Surgeon General:

> In past armed conflicts, the combat amputee has been a significant clinical problem for the military medical care system due to the severity of the injuries, the associated morbidity, and prolonged hospitalization. The likelihood of military operations using ground forces in landmine filled Afghanistan require [sic] proactive planning for multiple amputee casualties. The Russians reported on their experience in Afghanistan that in 1978 land mines accounted for 4% of all injuries—the rates in 80, 82, 84, and 86 were 8%[,] 18%[,] 21%[,] and 24%[,] respec-

---

[1]   Appendix A provides more context for battlefield amputations, including prior to 9/11.

tively, as the use of land mines proliferated. The time to medical treatment because of the mountainous terrain and transport difficulties was: under 6 hrs[,] 4% of patients received medical treatment (other than initial first aid); 6–12 hrs, 21%[;] 12–24 hrs 25%[;] 2 days or greater 50% of patients. (Scoville, 2001a, p. 1)

Within a matter of days, a team from OTSG and the WRAMC developed a plan for a new amputee center to provide for the "special care needed by amputees in the transition from a wounding to final prosthetic fitting, . . . before a patient is treated by the VA system" (McHale, 2001a, p. 2). They thought that such "amputee care requires a team approach of surgeons, nurses, therapists, psychiatrists, prosthetists, and social workers to help not only in the physical transformation of the patient but be able to provide vocational or other opportunities to make the amputee a productive member of society" (McHale, 2001b). They also suggested that "the most likely site for establishing a center for amputee care would be Walter Reed Army Medical Center," because it is "the most likely place for evacuation for an upcoming conflict" and "already has a modern brace and limb service that could easily be expanded" (McHale, 2001a, p. 2).

On October 31, 2001, the Army Surgeon General approved plans to develop a "virtual" amputee system in which the level of care would be consistent across the Army,[2] and to establish a care center at Walter Reed and a new course of instruction to train surgeons prior to deployment (Scoville, 2003d). By the beginning of December 2001, a panel of outside experts was developing "a consensus doctrine for the care of military amputee care from injury in theater to rehabilitation to return to duty/discharge, . . . space and patient flow at WRAMC for amputee care, . . . [and] available equipment . . . to verify ability to provide state of the art amputee care and identify additional requirements" (Scoville, 2001d).[3]

Unfortunately, the new system was not in place when the first amputees arrived (one in 2001, one in 2002, and in larger numbers beginning in 2003). Indicative of the way things had been, the first group of ten amputees stayed an average 51 days before being transferred to the VA, and "the majority of patients were discharged from outpatient care with a temporary prosthesis, physical therapy routines in pamphlet form, limited or no occupational therapy and the basic ability to ambulate independently in

---

[2]   The "virtual" system envisioned Walter Reed "at the center of a multi-site, coordinated complex of facilities that include regional medical centers in Europe, Brooke Army Medical Center in San Antonio, the Department of Veterans Affairs, and other military and civilian treatment facilities. Wherever in the virtual system that amputee patients receive care, the goal of the US Army Amputee Patient Care Program (USAAPCP) is to ensure that they receive the kind of care that will allow them to lead lives unconstrained by their amputation" (Scoville, 2004c, p. i).

[3]   Initial meetings took place at WRAMC on December 2–3, 2001, to identify requirements for amputee care and develop plans for managing light, medium, and heavy casualty loads. A second symposium for amputee care providers was held at Uniformed Services University of the Health Sciences (USUHS) on August 19, 2002, sponsored by WRAMC Department of Orthopaedics, again involving leaders in amputee care from both the civilian health care sector and the VA. See Scoville (2003c).

a wheelchair, crutches or initial prosthesis" (Scoville, 2006a). These outcomes were not consistent with the Army's vision for how to care for this patient population, and were in stark contrast to later outcomes, where patients often remained in treatment for a year or more while assigned to local medical hold commands, and where they received several definitive prosthetic devices for a variety of activities. We describe below how this system of care evolved and matured.

Building a New System of Care for the Combat Amputee

Planning went forward during the spring and summer of 2002, and on August 22, 2002, the Surgeon General gave final approval for Walter Reed to be the Army's primary site, with a capacity of ten acute inpatients and 50 long-term advanced-function outpatients; BAMC at Fort Sam Houston, Texas, was designated as the secondary site.[4] Initial funding for the program and for renovations to WRAMC ($2.5 million) was to come immediately from the Chief of Staff of the Army in 2002. Subsequently, appropriated funds from Congress included $2.4 million in fiscal year (FY) 2003, $10 million in FY 2004, $7.8 million in FY 2005, and $3.9 million in FY 2006 (Scoville, 2006a). In addition, an outside Amputee Care Program Board of Directors was established to "serve in an advisory capacity to broaden the scope of vision for the amputee care program, [and to] make such suggestions for the improvement of the program as it deems necessary" (U.S. Department of the Army, 2003b, p. 1; Doukas, 2003).

These new facilities were a marked change from Army centers established during previous wars in that they employed a team approach to care. Previously, service members with amputations received their care from a variety of different medical specialties that best met their immediate medical or surgical needs, and as a result "their holistic and amputee-specific care was less than consistent" (Pasquina et al., 2009, p. 8). At the WRAMC, a new Department of Orthopaedics and Rehabilitation was established to bring all critical subspecialties needed for the care of those with amputations (orthopaedics, physical medicine and rehabilitation, occupational therapy, physical therapy [PT], and prosthetics and orthotics) together into a single united department that followed a new patient flow protocol, working with a new set of team guidelines (Scoville, 2002a, 2002b) and taking a multidisciplinary approach to collaboratively provide rehabilitation to patients. Together with new technological advancements, the team approach spurred additional rehabilitative options for patients. We discuss two prominent advancements—prosthetic inventions and the Computer-Assisted Rehabilitation Environment (CAREN)—in Appendix B.

---

[4] See Scoville (2003c). BAMC amputee patient care site would have a formal opening ceremony on January 14, 2005, as noted in Scoville (2005c). The third location, Comprehensive Combat and Complex Casualty Care (C5) in San Diego, started seeing patients after the other two sites.

Implementation of the new team approach was facilitated by DOD's establishment of three advanced rehabilitation centers and a center of excellence for extremity trauma and amputation, discussed in the following sections.

Military Advanced Training Center at Walter Reed Army Medical Center

By the end of 2003, it was clear that existing rehabilitation facilities at Walter Reed were inadequate. A plan for short-term amputee patient care space requirements was initiated to alleviate the overcrowding. Specifically, a temporary pod was leased and installed on the tennis court to house routine PT care, but what was needed was a new free-standing clinic extension.[5] In November 2003, Congress asked the Army for an "infrastructure improvement plan for the United States Army Amputee Patient Care Program (USAAPCP) based at Walter Reed Army Medical Center in Washington, D.C."[6] On January 20, 2004, the *Infrastructure Improvement for the U.S. Army Amputee Patient Care Program* was submitted to Congress (Scoville, 2004c). The report called for a new Military Amputee Training Center (MATC) to be constructed at Walter Reed.

In the report to Congress the Army Surgeon General noted:

> The existing clinics at Walter Reed are designed for routine cases and workloads. They are inadequate for the large influx of amputee patients training to achieve military performance goals. New patients from Middle East operations are exceeding the capacity of the current program. Although a short-term solution to patient-care space has been initiated, a long-term solution is still urgently needed.
>
> The advanced clinical care, training and research protocols being developed by the USAAPCP demand specially designed space and equipment. Training to the highest levels of athleticism that is now possible requires numerous activities that build and test limits of the patient's strength, balance, agility and endurance.
>
> These facilities are embodied in the proposed Advanced Amputee Training Center. This specialized facility would be a first-of-its-kind hybrid of clinical care, research and athletic facilities providing advanced resources for fitting, testing and adjusting advanced prosthetics, for physical and occupational therapy; social work,

---

[5] Short-term options and alternatives were reviewed in Scoville (2003f).

[6] The House Record No. 108-401 of the FY 2004 Defense Omnibus Bill, from November 25, 2003, contained the following:

Walter Reed Amputee Center

The conferees are aware of Walter Reed Army Medical Center's efforts to improve amputee treatment and rehabilitation, especially in light of the growing number of injured military members returning from Operation Iraqi Freedom who require such care. As such, the conferees direct the Surgeon General of the Army to prepare and submit an infrastructure improvement plan for the Walter Reed Amputee Center to the congressional defense committees. The plan should be submitted not later than January 15, 2004, and should include a detailed description of the types of infrastructure improvements needed, a timetable for making these improvements, and associated cost estimates. (Scoville, 2007c)

psychology, clinical nutritional services, and clinical research. Advanced training areas include indoor walking, running and maneuver lanes, uneven terrain simulation areas, stairs and other obstacles and surface features, climbing surfaces and various specialized equipment and space for advanced strength, balance, agility and motor skill therapy. (Scoville, 2004c, p. ii)

The new center was projected to cost $10.9 million, of which $9.3 million was the cost of the actual construction of a 27,090-square-foot facility. The project was approved by Congress, and ground was broken for the new facility on November 19, 2004, but construction was delayed in part because of plans made in 2005 by the Defense Base Realignment and Closure (BRAC) Commission to close Walter Reed and co-locate the flagship Army facility with the Navy on the Navy's Bethesda, Maryland, campus. The new joint center would be called the Walter Reed National Military Medical Center (WRNMMC). As an interim measure, the Army Trauma Training Center (ATTC) was completed in 2007 at the old Walter Reed site and was to be used until 2011, when a new facility would be ready at the new joint WRNMMC, where amputee care was to be integrated into the PT and occupational therapy clinics in a free-standing structure.[7]

Today, the new joint center in Bethesda, designated the MATC, provides state-of-the-art care not only to combat service members with amputations, but also "Wounded, Ill and Injured Service Members, Retirees and Family Members [using] sophisticated prosthetics and cutting-edge athletic equipment to confirm pre-injury capabilities as they restore their sense of selves" (WRNMMC, undated).

Brooke Army Medical Center and the Center for the Intrepid

Building on the success of the MATC, in the spring of 2005, the family of Zachary and Elizabeth Fisher announced plans to raise $55 million for the construction of a world-class state-of-the-art physical rehabilitation facility, the Center for the Intrepid (CFI), at BAMC in San Antonio, Texas (Intrepid Fallen Heroes Fund, 2005; Scoville, 2005b).[8] The Army Surgeon General agreed (Scoville, 2005a), and the CFI was dedicated on January 29, 2007, along with a new Fisher House for families of hospitalized military personnel. The CFI had a staff of 55, including active duty Army medical staff, Department of the Army civilians, contract providers, and 9 full-time VA employees (Hooper, 2007).

---

[7] As discussed in Scoville (2005d), Scoville (2006b), Scoville (2006c), and Scoville (2007d).

[8] Zachary Fisher was a prominent real estate investor who founded the Intrepid Museum Foundation in 1979 to save the historic aircraft carrier USS *Intrepid*. In 1982, he started the Zachary and Elizabeth M. Fisher Armed Services Foundation for the construction and support of comfort homes for families of hospitalized military personnel; today 70 Fisher Houses operate at military bases and VA medical centers throughout the nation. After his death in 1999, his family continued its support for the military, and after 9/11, they established the Intrepid Fallen Heroes Fund as an independent nonprofit organization.

Comprehensive Combat and Complex Casualty Care Facility at Naval Medical Center San Diego

While the facility at Walter Reed cared primarily for Army patients, it also cared for Marines, Navy Air Force, and DOD civilian amputees (Scoville, 2004b). During a visit to Walter Reed, the Commandant of the Marine Corps asked why the Navy, which provided medical support for the Marine Corps, could not take care of the Marines. Soon after the Navy Surgeon General's Office began plans to establish a center for amputee care at the NMCSD, which would allow wounded Marines on the West Coast the opportunity to receive the same level of care closer to their home duty station at Camp Pendleton.[9] The Navy's Comprehensive Combat and Complex Casualty Care (C5) facility at the NMCSD received its first patient in October 2006 and was fully operational by October 2007. The C5 facility was designed to provide aesthetically and medically advanced prosthetic and rehabilitation services. Its "state of the art gait lab includes a high resolution, accurate motion capture system to digitally acquire, analyze and display three-dimensional motion data, [and] provide quantitative documentation of walking or running ability as well as identification of any underlying cause for gait deviations" (NMCSD, undated).

The Extremity Trauma and Amputation Center of Excellence

In 2009, Congress mandated the establishment of the EACE collaborative organization to enhance partnerships between DOD, the VA, institutions of higher education, and other appropriate public and private entities. As directed by Congress, the EACE undertakes activities to

> implement a comprehensive plan and strategy for the Department of Defense and the Department of Veterans Affairs; [and] conduct research to develop scientific information aimed at saving injured extremities, avoiding amputations, and preserving and restoring the function of injured extremities. . . . Such research . . . [also] address[es] military medical needs . . . include[ing] the full range of scientific inquiry encompassing basic, translational, and clinical research; [and carries] out such other activities to improve and enhance the efforts of the Department of Defense and the Department of Veterans Affairs for the mitigation, treatment, and rehabilitation of traumatic extremity injuries and amputations. (Public Law 110-417, 2008, Sect. 723)

Of particular note is the Clinical Affairs Division, which analyzes and disseminates

> standards of care and evidence-based practices and provides policy guidance for the treatment, management, and rehabilitation of extremity injuries and amputa-

---

[9]   As noted in Scoville (2006a). In May 2005, the Office of Administration at NMCSD started work on "a proposal paper for creating an amputee care center at Naval Medical Center San Diego" (Cherry, 2005).

tions in order to mitigate co-morbidities and maximize the functional return of patients. Determining best practices, particularly in the field of prosthetics, can bring about significant cost savings as well as enhance readiness by allowing service members to return to full duty. (EACE, undated)

The Research and Surveillance Division of EACE conducts clinically relevant research in support of the treatment, mitigation, and rehabilitation of amputation and limb trauma.

EACE consists of a headquarters that is split between San Antonio and Washington, D.C. Its staff, approximately 40 at the time of writing of this report, includes researchers, most of whom are clinicians, educators, and administrators. EACE does not manage the health care provider assets for whom this study is developing competencies; military treatment facility (MTF) commanders do. Beginning in FY 2019, as a result of the FY 2017 National Defense Authorization Act (NDAA) (Public Law 114-328, 2016), the Defense Health Agency (DHA) will operate garrison MTFs. Therefore, the results of this study will be important to each of these organizations.

A New Standard of Care for the Army: Redefining Medical Discharge and the Transfer of Patients to the Department of Veterans Affairs

Prior to 9/11, the ultimate responsibility for service members who had experienced amputation(s) belonged to the VA; afterward, the Army saw it quite differently. As the Chief of the Amputee Patient Care Center at Walter Reed explained,

> After previous military conflicts, soldiers who underwent an amputation typically received immediate life-saving medical treatment and limb stabilization in a military medical facility. Once a patient was stable, the trend was to medically discharge soldiers w/ amputations and transition them over to the Veteran's Administration healthcare system for rehabilitation and prosthetic care. After Operation Desert Storm, we realized that an amputation was not necessarily a career-ending injury, especially with the evolution of new prosthetics that allow soldiers to run, jump, etc. Now, after Operations Enduring Freedom and Iraqi Freedom, the military's attitude toward rehabilitation of the soldier/amputee has evolved into a proactive team-effort approach. The Walter Reed Army Medical Center has established the Amputee Center of Excellence. This center provides a full spectrum of state-of-the-art care for soldiers who sustain traumatic amputations on the battlefield. This team is dedicated to the rehabilitation and restoration of soldiers; the end goal is to provide soldiers the option to remain on/return to active duty and complete their military careers. (Scoville, 2003e, p. 1)

But it was more than just giving these patients the opportunity to return to active duty that was driving the new system. The Army saw that it had a role in the continued care for amputees even after they had left service, since amputees who were medically retired had access to the military health care system, if they chose to use it, for the rest of their lives. Moreover, the Army noted that "patients . . . may elect to continue their care at Walter Reed, or may seek additional care at facilities closer to their home. The amputee care program provides the opportunity for patients to return to WRAMC periodically for re-evaluation, revisions or refinements to their prosthetic devices, and an intensive rehabilitation program" (Polly, 2003, p. 1).

As the Army saw it:

> All of the individuals sustaining combat amputations are high-level athletes and the goal is to return them to the highest level of activity that they wish to achieve. These physiologically young individuals differ from the average amputees in the civilian sector who often are lower level activity patients that function well with basic prosthetic appliances.
>
> The standard of care on the civilian sector, and in the Veteran's Health Administration, is to return the amputee patient to a community ambulation level with capabilities to perform all activities of daily living. The standard of the US Army Amputee Patient Care Program is to return all individuals to the highest level of activity achievable. This includes running and ambulation on uneven terrain for the lower extremity amputee patient, and strenuous upper body activity, including overhead skills for the upper extremity amputee.
>
> It is projected that these patients will return to WRAMC on numerous occasions for advanced skills training and prosthetic enhancements. (Scoville, 2003b)

In the era of the all-volunteer force (AVF) the Army's goal is to "return each patient to the highest level of function possible" (Scoville, 2003f), or as the Army explained it in a report to Congress, "the goal of the USAAPCP [US Army Amputee Patient Care Program] is to return patients to their pre-injury level of activity, called 'tactical athleticism'" (Scoville, 2004c, p. 4–1). On December 18, 2003, President George W. Bush visited the Amputee Patient Center at Walter Reed and in prepared remarks said:

> Americans would be surprised to learn that a grievous injury, such as the loss of a limb, no longer means forced discharge. In other words, the medical care is so good and the recovery process is so technologically advanced, that people are no longer forced out of the military. When we're talking about forced discharge, we're talking about another age and another army. This is a new age, and this is a new army. Today if wounded service members want to remain in uniform and can do the job, the military tries to help them stay. (Bush, 2003)

In addition, amputees of today's AVF are generally medically retired and can select care provided by the VA or the Army, or both.

U.S. Army Wounded Warrior Program

To facilitate retaining amputees on active duty in April 2004, the Army initiated the Disabled Soldier Support System (DS3) program, which was renamed the U.S. Army Wounded Warrior Program (AW2) in November 2005. Its aim is to help "disabled soldiers cut through red tape to seek out the help or information they need until they can return to active duty or receive a medical retirement from the military" (Miles, 2004). The program provides "disabled soldiers a single starting point for help with their financial, administrative, medical, vocational and other needs. It also helps them sort out the medical and vocational entitlements and other benefits for which they qualify" (Miles, 2004). As envisioned, the program was to

> incorporate and integrate several existing programs to provide holistic support services for our severely disabled Soldiers and their families throughout their phased progression from initial casualty notification to their return to home station and final career position. DS3 will also use a system to track and monitor severely disabled Soldiers for up to five years beyond their medical retirements to provide appropriate assistance through an array of existing service providers. (*Staff of Soldiers Magazine*, 2005, p. 1)

To be eligible for the program, a wounded soldier needed to have a 30 percent or greater disability from a *single* cause. Technically, eligibility extended to soldiers with the following disabling conditions: "Blindness/Vision Loss; Amputation; Spinal Cord Injury and Paralysis; Severe Burns; Severe Hearing Loss/Deafness; Permanent Disfigurement; Traumatic Brain Injury (TBI); Post Traumatic Stress Disorder (PTSD); and/ or Fatal, Incurable Disease with Limited Life Expectancy" (Hudak et al., 2009, p. 567), but in practice the program, as the Director of the DS3 program emphasized, was limited to those casualties that involved paralysis or the loss of limbs or eyes. During the first year of the program (2004), 340 soldiers were eligible; of these, 179 were eligible because of a major limb amputation (Hudak et al., 2009; Carino, 2016b).

In 2008, eligibility for the program was changed to include "soldiers who have received, or are expected to receive, a 50 percent or higher combined disability rating from the Army because of combat or combat-related injuries" (Hudak et al., 2009, p. 567), and the number of soldiers in the program grew from 2,432 in 2007 to 4,329 by April 1, 2009, with most of the growth coming from soldiers suffering from PTSD and TBI.[10] Given the large number of soldiers reported to have PTSD, TBI, and major limb amputations,[11] the AW2 program was covering all major limb amputees, about 4

---

[10] The Army reported that on April 1, 2009, 4,329 soldiers were enrolled in the AW2 program: approximately, 1,300 with PTSD, 700 with TBI, and slightly fewer than 700 with amputations (Cheek, 2009).

[11] Between October 2001 and December 2008, the Army reported 33,198 cases of PTSD among soldiers who had been deployed to Afghanistan and Iraq; 2,489 cases of severe or penetrating TBI; and 671 soldiers who had a major limb amputation (Carino, 2016a).

percent of those with PTSD, and about 28 percent of those with "severe or penetrating" TBI.

Retaining Service Members with Amputation(s) on Active Duty

Given the goal to retain amputees on active duty, the success of the program and the rehabilitation of amputees can be seen in the unprecedented large number of amputees electing to continue on active duty. In the past, few soldiers who had a limb amputated remained on active duty. While there is a long history of invalid soldiers continuing to serve, amputees generally did not remain in active service (Kishbaugh et al., 1995). After Vietnam, several who remained made significant contributions, including now-retired General Frederick Franks, a transtibial amputee who commanded the VII Corps during Operation Desert Storm, and former Chief of Staff of the Army, General Eric Shinseki, a partial-foot amputee (Scales, 1993). It was General Shinseki who provided the initial funds to support the USAAPCP at Walter Reed.

Generally, service members who have experienced amputation(s) are considered unfit for military service, but the discharge process is a lengthy and, at times, confusing process, especially insofar as it involves determining the service member's fitness for service and, in most cases, level of disability. At the time the USAAPCP was established, Army Regulation 40-501 (U.S. Department of the Army, 2003a) directed that amputees of the upper or lower extremities be referred to a medical evaluation board (MEB) for evaluation of their condition. Given the new emphasis on retaining as many amputees to active service as practical, the regulation was changed,[12] and amputees were given a "temporary profile," which allowed them to remain in rehabilitation for additional weeks or months so they might achieve a higher level of function, including the ability to perform pertinent military skills. Now, if a service member achieves the maximum medical benefit from care in less than one year and there is no longer a projected ability to improve the service member's condition, or if the service member reaches one year on a temporary profile, he or she is referred to the MEB. In a few cases, service members who have experienced amputation(s) have been able to demonstrate that they can fully meet all the physical requirements of their military occupations and are found "fit for duty" during the MEB or physical evaluation board (PEB). In such cases, the soldier is assigned to a job appropriate for his or her rank and skills.

In most cases, the PEB finds the service member is not fit for duty, at which point he or she may request a continuance on active duty (COAD) waiver, which is normally granted since the amputation occurred as a result of combat, if the soldier can "dem-

---

[12] Chapter 3 of Army Regulation 40-501, which describes how soldiers with significant limb loss are to be evaluated, was changed to provide that "Soldiers with amputations will (assuming no other disqualifying medical conditions) be provided a temporary profile not less than 4 months (but not to exceed 1 year) to enable the Soldier to attain maximum medical benefit" (Department of the Army, 2007, p. 24).

Figure 2.1
Retention on Active Duty of Army Major Limb Amputees: October 2001–April 2016

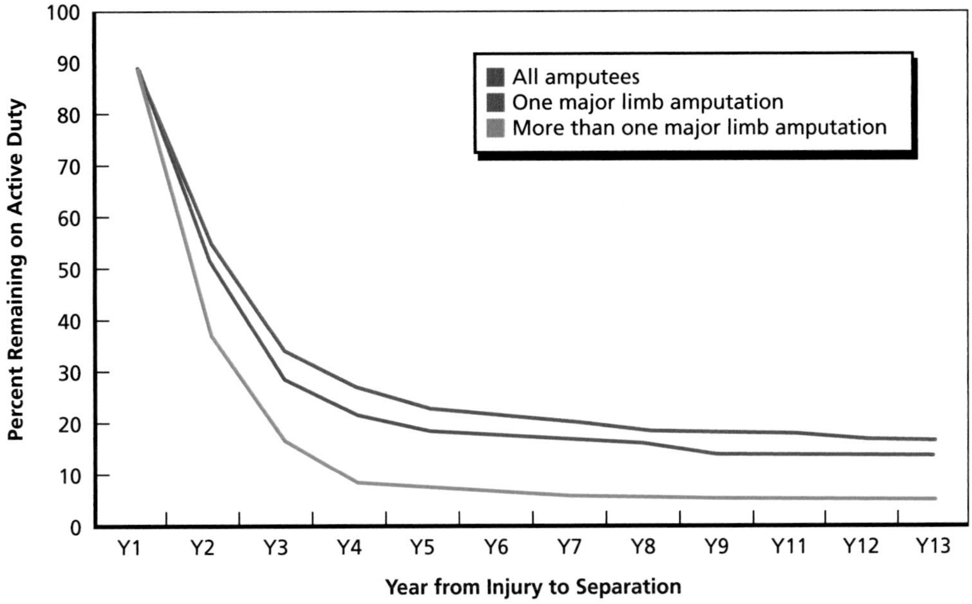

SOURCE: Carino, 2016b.

onstrate a higher level of function with a prosthesis and have the recommendation of two medical officers" (Stinner et al., 2010, p. 1476). An analysis of 395 combat-related major limb amputations between October 1, 2001, and June 1, 2006, showed that 65 amputees (16.5 percent) remained on active duty, 11 were "fit for duty," and 54 received COAD waivers. These results are consistent with more recent data presented in Figure 2.1, which shows longer-term retention of 14 percent for all amputees; 17 percent for amputees who lost one limb; and 5 percent for amputees who lost more than one limb. The retention of 17 percent for all amputees, however, is somewhat lower than what the USAAPCP once considered possible, which was that "nearly 40 percent of patients could reach a level of function necessary to return to active duty military service if they so choose" (Scoville, 2004a). In other words, a little less than half the service members with amputation(s) who at one time were considered physically retainable actually continue serving.

This chapter has described how care for service members with deployment-related amputation(s) has evolved since 9/11, through the construction of state-of-the-art facilities and a center of excellence, as well as a shift in how the Army views the ability of these service members to continue to serve. We now turn to the services involved in the provision of rehabilitation and the competencies individual providers need to continue to provide these rehabilitative opportunities to patients.

CHAPTER THREE

Developing a Competency Model: Interviews and Technical Expert Surveys

In this chapter, we describe the methodology used to develop core competencies, and we then present the findings. Our approach consisted of interviews and a TES, which we describe in the next two sections.

Patient, Provider, and Subject Matter Expert Interviews

As mentioned in Chapter One, one of our objectives was to identify the types of services and providers that are integral to amputation rehabilitation. To do so, we conducted semistructured phone and in-person interviews with patients, subject matter experts, and a wide range of health care providers to understand their perspectives about a variety of topics besides the services that were integral to optimal care for patients who have experienced amputation(s). These topics included the most relevant behaviors needed to rehabilitate that patient population, areas where skill atrophy might occur and ways to overcome such atrophy, and best practices they perceived in military treatment facilities. While some feedback we received was oriented toward clinical behaviors (e.g., how to don/doff a liner and a prosthesis), much of what we aimed to learn during our interviews could be characterized as administrative and organizational. In part, this was intentional. We assume that providers have met the clinical requirements of their profession and the facility where they are employed, as demonstrated by privileges and credentials. We framed the interview questions around five of the seven phases of care included in the Amputee Coalition's Rehabilitation Process framework (see Figure 1.2): postoperative, preprosthetic, preparatory prosthetic training, definitive prosthetic training, and reintegration. The interview guides for DOD providers and patients/family members are contained in Appendix C.[1]

---

[1] Both guides were created to facilitate semistructured interviews. Questions were tailored as the interview progressed and we learned more about the respondent's experiences, as well as rephrased if the language in the guide was too technical or not precisely relevant to the subject.

Most health care providers we interviewed currently worked at one of three DOD facilities: MATC, CFI, or C5. We also interviewed patients/family members who had received rehabilitation services at one of these sites. When we were preparing for our visits, we recruited interview participants in a variety of ways. In some cases, a point of contact (POC) at the installation contacted staff to notify them of our visit and to solicit volunteers, whom we then emailed with an invitation to be interviewed. For some visits, a POC on-site worked directly with staff prior to the visit to create an interview schedule, and we made ourselves available for anyone who was interested in being interviewed (scheduled in advance or available day-of). We did not have precise information on the total number of providers who could be interviewed, so we recruited and interviewed all providers for whom we had contact information or who showed up in our interview room. In total, we interviewed 27 patients/family members and 85 health care providers who provide one of the services listed in Table 3.1. There is considerable variation in the number of interviewees by service area, which is due primarily to differences in underlying staff numbers. For example, there are many more occupational and PTs than there are recreational therapists (included in our "other" category). That is because most of the occupational therapists see patients in other diagnostic groups (so more of them are needed on staff to be able to accommodate more patients), whereas recreational therapists generally work specifically with patients who have had amputations. Table 3.1 contains the number of interviews we conducted for each service, as well as the number of full-time equivalents (FTEs) for each working at MATC, CFI, or C5 as of May 2018.

We analyzed the interview transcripts in Dedoose, which is an application that allows one to process interview and other qualitative data. As we reviewed the initial transcripts, multiple team members coded the same interview to ensure that the coding was being done consistently, and multiple transcripts were coded to ensure consistency across transcripts. Once the codebook was finalized (see Appendix D), we applied it to all transcripts; each transcript was coded by one member of the research team. The codebook provided an organizing framework for us to highlight important themes related to the phases of care being described by the interviewee, roles/tasks and knowledge/skills described by the interviewee, and other issues mentioned during the interviews. We then clustered similar roles/tasks and their underlying knowledge/skills into groups, which we labeled as being indicative of a competency. Team members discussed the label or name of each competency, which turned into the initial set of competencies. As part of the competency discussion, we identified exemplar behaviors that aligned with KSAOs noted for the different competencies. Exemplar behaviors were derived from interviews, literature, and site visits. The competencies and exemplar behaviors were, in turn, presented in our TES, which is described next.

Table 3.1
Number of Interviews Conducted

Service	Number of Interviews	Full-Time Equivalents (May 2018)
Behavioral Health	5	5.5
Case Management	4	n/a
Diet and Nutrition	5	0.5
Occupational Therapy	11	11
Orthopaedic Surgery	8	n/a
Physical Therapy	22	17.25
Physical Medicine and Rehabilitation	5	3.1
Prosthetics and Orthotics	7	17.5
Biomedical Engineering	8	n/a
Patients	27	
Other	10	

NOTES: The number of FTEs can be smaller than the total number of individual providers. For example, the 3.1 physical medicine and rehabilitation FTEs represent five individual providers: 0.5 FTEs at MATC, 0.1 FTE at C5, and two full-time providers, plus one provider working halftime, at CFI. The relationship between FTEs and individuals providers was clear for behavioral health but not for all services, according to the data call conducted by EACE in May 2018. This relationship, in addition to the fact that there may have been attrition in staffing since the interviews were conducted, explains why some interview counts are greater than the number of May 2018 FTEs. Case management, orthopaedic surgery, and biomedical engineering were not part of the data call.

Technical Expert Surveys

The technical expert survey phase of this research involved several steps, with the ultimate goals of (1) developing a single competency framework for the set of services studied, which would be relevant for guiding rehabilitative care for service members who experienced deployment-related extremity amputations, and (2) identifying a set of behaviors for each type of service that is representative of each competency.

Approach

We first developed an overarching competency framework that was used to organize skills, behaviors, and knowledge (described in more detail below). This framework was developed based on a review of some of the competency frameworks described in Chapter One; specifically, we relied on the IOM competency framework for health care professionals (Institute of Medicine, 2003) as well as competency frameworks from discipline-specific professional organizations and accrediting bodies (e.g., Accreditation Council for Graduate Medical Education; American Occupational Therapy Association; Council on Social Work Education), and we tailored these to the amputation rehabilitation context based on the interviews described in the previous section. Our conceptualization of a competency is consistent with DOD's Competency Management Framework, given that we focused on "observable, measurable pattern[s] of knowledge skills and abilities" that "include behaviors associated with job performance" (DOD, 2016, p. 15).

We used a modified Delphi approach to develop the TES. We designed the TES to collect ratings on behaviors as well as KSAOs needed for providing quality care for patients with amputation(s) and to measure consensus on the items. The TES included two rounds of online surveys in which experts within each service category rated the skills, behaviors, and knowledge (referred to collectively as *behaviors*) required for providing quality amputee care. Typically, competency modeling or job analysis would involve two independent groups of experts, but we asked the same group of experts to respond to both rounds of our survey. The reason for this is twofold. Our original intent was to have a live discussion with all experts for each provider group, but scheduling challenges prohibited that. This modified Delphi approach allowed for a virtual "discussion," because the same individuals were able to respond in the round two survey to comments provided during the first round. Second, because the population of providers within DOD for each service was small, and because we wanted to include as many DOD experts as possible, it would not have been feasible to identify enough participants for two independent groups of experts.

To develop the surveys, the first step was to identify a set of related behaviors associated with quality rehabilitation following amputation. We focused our review of behaviors on three sources: (1) existing competency frameworks and/or practice standards for each discipline; (2) relevant information from *Care of the Combat Amputee* (Lenhart, Pasquina, and Cooper, 2009); and (3) interviews with providers and subject matter experts during site visits and telephone calls. The study team identified relevant KSAOs and developed a comprehensive list by service. If there were two items that were similar in nature but had varying degrees of detail, we combined them into a single item to avoid duplication. On the other hand, when two different behaviors were combined in a single item, such as providing inpatient and outpatient care, we separated it into two individual behaviors to ensure we received a response for each.

Next, the complete list of behaviors was organized into the proposed competency framework by three researchers to confirm consistency across services TES. Behaviors that could potentially fit into multiple competencies were reviewed by a fourth researcher and discussed until consensus was reached.

Last, the TESs were programmed into a series of online surveys (using Select Survey) by rehabilitative service and tested by two researchers prior to fielding. Experts were emailed a link to the survey, information about the study, and a description of the purpose and goal of the survey.[2] Respondents included providers who participated in the study qualitative interviews,[3] providers recommended by EACE, and providers who worked in the VA or civilian settings identified through online searches and literature. Our aim was to have at least four respondents per survey; therefore, we invited at least ten respondents in each service category.[4]

Data Collection
First Round Survey

Surveys were administered in two rounds. Drawing on procedures often used in job analytic frameworks,[5] the first round asked experts to rate the frequency and importance of each behavior using the following scales and response options:

- Frequency: How often do you apply this knowledge, skill, ability, or behavior when caring for amputees?[6]
  - Response options: always, often, sometimes, rarely, never.
- Importance: How important is this knowledge, skill, ability, or behavior to providing quality care to amputees?

---

[2] We invited both DOD and civilian experts to participate in the TESs. Because our surveys drew on the information collected during interviews, we aimed to invite providers who were not interviewed. In some cases, there simply were not enough DOD providers who hadn't been interviewed who could be invited to participate in a TES, primarily due to the broad reach extended to conduct enough interviews to identify competencies (five interviews were required). We prioritized conducting at least five interviews by service area, which resulted in not always having enough DOD providers for the TES. However, in the same way that we wanted to learn about best practices at civilian rehabilitation centers, we also saw value in inviting civilians who are experts in their field. DOD recommends that the experts who validate competencies should work in the environment where the competencies will be used. In that sense, our TESs serve only as an initial validation of our competencies and behaviors. Our recommendations, which appear in the final chapter of this report, address validation among DOD experts.

[3] We aimed to invite experts to the TES who were not interviewed previously. When we had difficulty reaching the minimum number of TES participants, either due to low underlying sample sizes or low response rates, we did invite individuals who were also invited to interview. We do not know how much overlap there was because we did not keep track of who was interviewed, but we expect that the number of individuals who participated in both an interview and a TES to be very small.

[4] As described below, we used a 70 percent threshold for agreement on the survey, which could be accomplished if three out of four experts agreed (but would not be reached by two out of three experts if we had a minimum of three). In addition, as shown in Table 3.1, the number of health care providers in DOD treating these patients (usually at the three advanced rehabilitation centers) is small, so it was not feasible to set a high minimum on the number of expert responses.

[5] See, for example, Drauden (1988, 2009).

[6] Note that for Behavioral Health and Prosthetist/Orthotist (the first two surveys), a slightly different version of this question was used. We asked, "How frequently does someone in your profession use this knowledge, skill, ability, or behavior?" The phrasing was revised in response to participant and team-member feedback.

- Response options: critically important, very important, moderately important, slightly important, not important.

In addition to rating the frequency and importance of each behavior, experts were asked to identify additional behaviors that were not reflected in the survey, but that they felt to be important for quality rehabilitation. Finally, experts were asked to provide feedback on the competency framework, including the terminology and definitions used to describe each competency.

When each survey closed we analyzed the data and calculated the proportion of responses for each behavior. The frequency and importance responses were combined into three groups for the purpose of identifying items that had consensus, which is consistent with how this has been done in the literature:[7]

- Frequency responses: always or often, sometimes, rarely or never.
- Importance responses: critically or very important, moderately important, slightly important

We analyzed the proportion of responses to calculate whether each behavior was low versus high importance and low versus high frequency, as well as examining the level of agreement between experts. We measured consensus using a threshold of 70 percent agreement for each service (Coleman, Hudson, and Maine, 2013). If at least 70 percent of experts consistently rated importance and frequency with the same response for a given behavior, it was identified as "high agreement." High and low agreement does not indicate direction of the response (e.g., whether something is critically important versus not at all important), but reflects consensus in the responses.

Second Round Survey

The second round of the survey asked the same experts from round one to rerate behaviors that had less than 70 percent agreement (or low agreement) in the first round survey. This practice is typical of a modified Delphi approach, in which the goal is to have the same respondents reflect on findings across two time points so that they can consider additional information before providing final ratings (Clay-Williams and Braithwaite, 2009; Janke et al., 2016; Sasahara et al., 2009).We created a summary of these items, including the proportions of individuals who provided ratings within each category for both frequency and importance, and included anonymous substantive feedback experts used during the first survey. The feedback was included to mimic a group conversation and allow experts to understand the ratings, feedback, and rationale of their peers. As part of this survey, experts were also asked to rate the proposed behaviors from the first round survey.

---

[7] See, for example, Janke et al. (2016); Sasahara et al. (2009).

Data Analysis

After the completion of the round two survey, we calculated the mean importance and frequency rating for each behavior by assigning a numerical score to the frequency and importance scales (importance scale ranged from 1, not important, to 5, critically important; frequency scale ranged from 1, never, to 5, always). Then, we calculated a weighted criticality score, which combines the frequency and importance ratings into a single score. Frequency and importance ratings are often combined into weighted criticality scores (Stutsky, Singer, and Renaud, 2012); for this study, we used an industry standard formula, which was: (importance × 2 + frequency). Using the weighted criticality score, another common industry practice, we organized the behaviors from highest to lowest score within each competency. The behaviors were also categorized as high and low agreement based on the second round survey. The criticality score was based on responses for items that reached the threshold of high agreement in the first survey and responses for the items that were rerated in the round two survey.

We originally planned to field both surveys for four to five weeks, but revised the schedule due to low response rates for some services. On a few occasions, we extended the deadline up to two weeks to reach our goal of at least four respondents (we set a minimum of three), and we sent at least two reminders for each round of surveys. To the extent possible, we aimed to receive responses from the same experts in the first and second surveys. Table 3.2 displays the number of responses we received for each service for each round of survey.

Table 3.2
Number of Responses to Technical Expert Surveys

Service	Number of Responses to First Survey	Number of Responses to Second Survey
Behavioral Health	5	5
Case Management	4	4
Diet and Nutrition	4	3
Occupational Therapy	4	3
Orthopaedic Surgery	5	3
Physical Therapy	8	3
Physical Medicine and Rehabilitation	6	3
Prosthetics and Orthotics	5	4
Biomedical Engineering	5	4

Core Competencies for Amputation Rehabilitation

As described previously, our initial framework was based on competency frameworks from the National Academies of Sciences (NAS), Engineering, and Medicine and discipline-specific professional organizations and accrediting bodies, as well as our provider interviews. Accordingly, an initial set of five competencies was identified: teamwork; teaching patients and family; military cultural awareness; patient-centered care; and evidence-based practice. In the process of reviewing behaviors across services, we made two revisions to the competency framework. First, several behaviors that related to cultural competence more generally (e.g., with respect to race, gender) emerged; therefore, we expanded the military cultural awareness category to reflect military and other cultural awareness. Second, several behaviors related to following ethical guidelines and understanding the laws and institutional policies that govern practice did not fit within the existing categories. Consequently, we created a sixth competency, which is also consistent with the frameworks of many professional organizations: ethical and professional behavior. The final RAND Arroyo Center competency framework for amputation rehabilitation appears in Figure 3.1.

For the purposes of the survey, we developed working definitions of each competency based in part on existing competency frameworks. However, we also asked participants for feedback on the framework. After refining the initial description of each competency based on this feedback, we propose the following definitions:

- **Teamwork** reflects the nature of interactions among members of the care team. This includes one-on-one consultation among providers and collaboration among providers.
- **Patient and family education** reflects the importance of providing education to patients and family members during the rehabilitation process.
- **Military and other cultural awareness** reflects factors related to cultural competence, including military cultural awareness and awareness of other cultural factors (e.g., ethnic, religious, gender).
- **Patient-centered care** reflects the importance of providing care that is responsive to the individual patient preferences and needs.
- **Evidence-based practice** reflects the importance of having knowledge of the scientific foundation of the field, as well as providing evidence-based and evidence-informed care. This includes best practices, clinical skill, and technical skill.
- **Ethical and professional behavior** reflects considerations related to ethical and professional behavior and includes behavior consistent with laws, policies, and regulations governing practice.

As described above, the purpose of the expert surveys was to identify a set of critical activities representative of each competency. As a result, we provided survey respon-

Figure 3.1
RAND Arroyo Center Competencies for Deployment-Related Amputation Rehabilitation

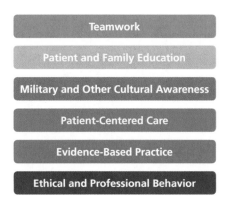

dents with the above definitions of each competency to make it easier for them to identify additional activities. The next section focuses on exemplar behaviors for these competencies.

Physical Therapy Behaviors for Amputation Rehabilitation

For the purposes of illustrating the results of the TESs, we present the findings for PTs, along with some sample quotations from PT interviews. As described above, after the two rounds of surveys were complete, we had ratings for each of the original activities included on the survey, as well as for new items that were proposed during the round one survey. The results tables for all services appear in Appendix E and contain all items developed and used in the surveys.

Each table in the appendix presents behaviors within each of the six competencies described above, as well as the mean importance, mean frequency, and weighted criticality scores for each of the behaviors, with behaviors sorted according to weighted critical score (with highest scores appearing first). In addition, we highlight in each table which behaviors reached consensus after the two rounds of surveys (labeled "high agreement" in the table), as well as those for which there was still a lack of agreement (labeled "low agreement").

Within the **teamwork** category, many items had high criticality scores, which is consistent with the expert interviews. The interviews identified the PT as a key member of the rehabilitation team, and the high criticality behaviors highlight the importance of collaboration, consultation, and cooperation with the rehabilitation team and effective communication skills. When explaining what happens when a patient requests an elective amputation, one PT described how the entire care team meets to present concerns, set expectations, and form a plan:

And that's where the team comes in. We all sit down and talk like "this is what I'm seeing." "Well, you're seeing that because this stuff's going on." "Oh, okay, well then maybe." We have discussions to say whether or not this is a good candidate and if it is, there is a border line. It's not uncommon for the team to get together with the patients and say, "Okay these are our concerns. This is what you need to do postoperatively if we're going to do this, are you going to do this?" And just lay it out. (Interview with physical therapy staff member, San Antonio, TX, CFI_PT_2 [name withheld on request])

All of the behaviors within the **patient and family education** category received high criticality scores as well. These behaviors highlight the role of PTs in teaching patients how to use and care for their prosthesis; teaching rehabilitation exercises; and educating patients and family members as to the goals of rehabilitation. These behaviors highlight that the role of PTs is critical across the phases of care—from the initiation of rehabilitation through the reintegration phase, in which they are preparing patients to be able to return to work and other activities. In addition, during the round one survey, respondents suggested additional items that are specific to the amputation rehabilitation context within this category and that reached a high level of agreement in round two. These include educating the patient on the appropriate fit of a prosthesis and how to don and doff a liner and prosthesis. There were also some items that were suggested that did not reach the threshold of high agreement, such as educating the patient on the management of sweat and on appropriate adaptive clothing. The comments provided by respondents on this item suggested that some perceived these tasks as within their scope, whereas others perceived them as falling more within the role of other service providers (e.g., PM&R, occupational therapy). One PT described how education is integral to everything they do with the patient and the importance of a consistent message coming from the entire care team:

Education is . . . people mention it but most of us don't talk about it that much because it's not separate from anything. I mean this is something that you start from the first time. . . . My first introduction, when I first meet a patient, we are starting to educate, especially amputees. Because there's so much stuff that they go through that is just absolutely foreign. . . . We know what's going to happen as they go through these phases as clinicians because we see it all the time. Well, that guy that's . . . he's the only person in the world to him that's ever gone through this. If we are not being very deliberate with our education, and making sure that our education when we are talking about this stuff is the same throughout the team. It's a singular message, which is another reason why the multidisciplinary team, the multidisciplinary meetings are so important. (Interview with physical therapy staff member, San Antonio, TX, CFI_PT_2 [name withheld on request])

Regarding **Military and other cultural awareness,** experts agreed that PTs must be comfortable touching a residual limb—a specific cultural aspect of providing care following an amputation. One PT explained:

> In my experience, when we were really hot in the war, it was like all day every day. Just getting guys to look at their leg for the first time. I would say during the period of, let's say 2006 to maybe 2010, 80 percent of my amputees that I took care of, I was probably the first one to unwrap their leg and let them really sit up, see it, touch it, and I think that's a huge part that PT plays along with the rest of the group. (Interview with physical therapy staff member, San Antonio, TX, CFI_PT_3 [name withheld on request])

They also endorsed the need to understand the unique preferences of the military patient population. However, there was not consensus on the use of the orthopaedic sports medicine model to return service members to optimal levels of functioning. Although this theme came up often during interviews, one survey respondent noted that this may not always be within the scope of the PT's job (and instead be within the scope of an adaptive trained personal trainer), while another indicated that a sports medicine model may not be the most appropriate, given an individual patient's goals or desires.

Regarding **patient-centered care,** all behaviors received high criticality ratings. These behaviors highlight the importance of being creative and flexible in problem-solving to meet an individual's rehabilitation needs; collaborating with the patient and family members to set goals; and developing rapport and a good working relationship with the patient. One PT described how to engage with a patient who is struggling with motivation:

> I think first, just sitting down with them and finding out what's going on with them and then what they do want. What their goals are and then just helping them work with either their therapist, work with the team to make sure that we're doing what they want. That we're helping them to be able to get to the level that they want to be at. Some people don't like . . . we push people, I think sometimes to walk. These really high amputees and stuff. I know I've seen some of them struggle and struggle. They're never gonna walk. They're not gonna be walkers because it's just too hard. For them, that's not their goal. Maybe there's other things that we should be concentrating on. (Interview with physical therapy staff member, San Antonio, TX, WR_PT_3 [name withheld on request])

Regarding **evidence-based practice**, some of the highly rated items describe the importance of integrating the best scientific evidence and staying current on best practices within PT. In addition, during the round one survey, respondents suggested several new items for which there was high agreement in the round two survey. Many of these were more specific to the context of amputation rehabilitation and included applying an understanding of available functional outcomes measures and then selecting the most appropriate measure for the patient, as well as understanding how prostheses work. However, several of the items that were specific to the amputation rehabilitation context did not reach a high level of agreement (e.g., understanding which muscles to lengthen and which to strengthen to provide the most symmetrical gait patterns); though respondents did not always provide a rationale for their ratings, the lack of agreement may reflect differences across settings.

Finally, the three behaviors in the **ethical and professional** practice category all received high criticality scores. These reflected the importance of practicing in a safe manner, practicing within the bounds of one's competence, and managing personal stress and reactions to patients.

The results tables for the other services appear in Appendix E.

Comparisons Across Service Categories

The results of the expert surveys provide important insight into the behaviors that are critical for the provision of quality rehabilitation following an amputation for each service. However, it is also instructive to review commonalities in the critical behaviors within competencies *across* services. Doing so may assist in the development of training or educational materials that will be relevant to a broader audience of services.

In reviewing behaviors across services, we found similarities within two competencies: teamwork and patient-centered care. An example of similar behaviors within the teamwork competency across service categories appears in Table 3.3. Though the wording varies from service to service, all of these behaviors highlight interactions with other health care providers, interpersonal and communication skills, and/or collaboration.

Table 3.3
Teamwork Behaviors Across Disciplines

Service	Behaviors
Behavioral Health	Use empathy, reflection, and interpersonal skills to effectively engage with other health professionals and members of the rehabilitation team
Physical Therapy	Apply interpersonal and communication skills to interactions with other providers
Prosthetics/Orthotics	Collaborate with other team members to develop medical and rehabilitation care plans
PM&R	Use interpersonal and communication skills that result in the effective exchange of information and collaboration with health professionals

Similarly, there was some consistency in patient-centered care behaviors across service categories. An example appears in Table 3.4. For each of these services, there were behaviors emphasizing the importance of understanding the specific needs, priorities, and goals of the patient; collaborating with the patient; and developing the treatment plan based on these components.

Table 3.4
Patient-Centered Care Behaviors Across Disciplines

Service	Behavior
Occupational Therapy	Collaborate with the client to develop and implement the intervention plan, on the basis of the client's needs and priorities, safety issues, and relative benefits and risks of the interventions
Case Management	Identify immediate, short-term, long-term, and ongoing needs, as well as develop appropriate and necessary case management strategies and goals to address those needs
Behavioral Health	Develop mutually agreed-on intervention goals and objectives based on the critical assessment of strengths, needs, and challenges with the patient
Physical Therapy	Establish and monitor a plan of care in consultation, cooperation, and collaboration with the patient/client

In addition, it is worth highlighting the results related to military and other cultural awareness. The behaviors in this category often received somewhat lower criticality ratings than the behaviors in teamwork and patient-centered care, and there was not always agreement within the group of experts as to the importance of behaviors in this category. However, there was at least some degree of consensus, particularly with respect to understanding aspects of military culture. Table 3.5 provides an example of behaviors related to military cultural awareness. Though military cultural awareness was found to be critical for PTs, occupational therapists, and case managers, the aspect of military culture that is relevant varies by profession. For physical and occupational therapists, it is key to understand the needs and preferences that military service members have with regard to rehabilitation (e.g., their rehabilitation goals). This reflects the role that these providers have in directing the focus of rehabilitation. However, for case managers, it is critical to understand military benefits, such as VA benefits, TRICARE insurance, and retirement disability—a behavior that reflects the role of case managers in coordinating care.

Table 3.5
Military and Other Cultural Awareness Behaviors Across Disciplines

Service	Behavior
Occupational Therapy and Physical Therapy	Understand the unique needs and preferences of a military patient population with regard to rehabilitation
Case Management	Demonstrate knowledge of VA, TRICARE/Medicare insurance, coverage levels, retirement disability, and other military-specific benefits

These examples highlight some of the similarities in behaviors across service categories. However, in other competencies, there was less cross-service consistency. For example, the evidence-based practice competency is an area in which the behaviors tended to be more specific to a given service. While most noted the importance of science-informed practice or providing care in a manner that reflects the current standards of practice, specific behaviors also reflected the roles and knowledge of each provider, such as psychological assessment for behavioral health or prosthesis technology for providers who fit patients with prosthetics. Therefore, training related to evidence-based practice would likely need to be tailored to a given service area. In this regard, experts have called into question whether evidence-based practice is equivalent to best practice, where the acceptance of the latter in organizational settings depends on broader contextual elements consistent with the way an organization is designed to deliver health care (Driever, 2002).

Additional Interview Findings

Our interview findings also helped us understand additional issues related to competencies, including concerns providers shared about skill atrophy and best practices currently used in DOD settings.

Atrophy

The three main concerns they mentioned as well as potential mitigation strategies included the need to

- document procedural steps before knowledge is lost.
  - For example, an orthotist recommended documenting steps in the fabrication process so that others would know about these steps.
- have providers share knowledge with others before they retire.
  - Providers noted that knowledge and skills are lost if not properly transmitted to staff still providing rehabilitative services.
- have opportunities to practice skills on patients as patient volume decreases.

- Multiple provider types recommended opening up services to other trauma patients (motorcycle accidents and in some cases oncology patients) because trauma patients provide opportunities for working with complex patients who are more similar to combat patients. As one provider noted, "I don't think there's a better way to do it. It's the only way to do it. The only way you get good at treating trauma is seeing trauma patients."
- Conversely, a prosthetist noted that disaster relief operations do not provide a good substitute for combat patients because it is difficult to wash the liner every day and replace componentry in disaster situations.
- In some cases, such as device repair, providers noted that seeing existing patients again can help ameliorate skill decline.

Best Practices

DOD providers also shared perspectives about what they viewed as best practices in DOD facilities. The main ones noted were

- a multidisciplinary team approach used by providers to communicate about patient progress and needs (as in an "amputee clinic," where a member of each provider/service attended to provide needed information about a patient's care plan).
- the co-location of providers in the same building (e.g., CFI) to facilitate the multidisciplinary approach.
- not having resource/reimbursement constraints in order to provide best rehabilitation services possible, including creating and/or procuring devices for patients
- having in-house prosthetists to allow for more efficient consults/collaboration with prosthetists.
- technological offerings (i.e., CAREN, fire-arm training simulator [FATS]) to help facilitate rehabilitation.
- support groups for patients and family members/spouses.

Summary

The results of these expert surveys provide important information about the competencies necessary to provide quality rehabilitation to individuals who have experienced amputation. Understanding these competencies—and the behaviors representative of these competencies—has a number of potential implications. First, these results can be used as the basis for training, education, and professional development opportunities for providers working with this population. An examination of the behaviors relevant to each competency within a service area could inform service-specific trainings or resources; these could include, for example, educational modules or decision tools that review available outcome measures and guide providers such as PTs to select the best outcome measure for a given patient. An examination of the behaviors that were similar across services, such as those related to teamwork or providing patient-centered care, may reveal opportunities to do cross-disciplinary trainings. For example, this could include a workshop regarding the best ways to assess an individual's rehabilitation preferences, needs, and goals, and how to use these to develop a patient-centered rehabilitation plan.

Though it was outside the scope of the present study, a next step in this competency modeling approach is to identify various levels of competence within each behavior or competency—for example, behaviors that would be expected of a novice versus an expert provider. Expanding on our results in this way would allow for the development of competency assessments with specific behavioral anchors for each level. Nonetheless, our TESs did provide initial evidence for the validity of the competencies and behaviors we identified from the literature and our interviews. Future work is needed to collect additional evidence of validity by examining the applicability of the competency model to the performance of current workforce members.

CHAPTER FOUR

Best Practices in Civilian Amputee Care for DOD Consideration

We also sought to understand best practices that civilian rehabilitation sites use when rehabilitating those who have experienced amputations. To accomplish this, we had two-person RAND Arroyo Center teams visit four of the highest-ranked civilian rehabilitation sites: the Shirley Ryan AbilityLab (formerly Rehabilitation Institute of Chicago), ranked #1 in the United States; The Institute for Rehabilitation and Research [TIRR] Memorial Hermann, ranked #2; Spaulding Rehabilitation Hospital, ranked #4; and the Shepherd Center, ranked #9 ("Best Hospitals," undated). These visits included tours of facilities and discussions with providers as well as leaders to understand how they care for those with amputations and approaches they use that might be indicative of best practices.

The best practices, standard of care, and core competencies for amputee care in the DOD may reflect care for the most traumatic forms of injury that people can survive. The characteristics of service-connected injury and trauma are less common in civilian health care facilities, but not without incident.

Civilian rehabilitation hospitals are a comparative setting where health care providers are managing the care of patients with traumatic injuries including amputations. We also studied civilian centers for specialty rehabilitative care to understand alternative perspectives to the health care challenge that DOD faces during peacetime operations, when there is a decline in the amount of traumatic injuries to military service members.

In this chapter, we present our findings from our visits to the highly ranked civilian centers in the United States. We summarize their health care delivery practices, key concerns for their health care providers, and potential best practices of relevance to DOD. The following is a high-level list of potential best practices for DOD to consider based on what the teams learned during civilian site visits, each of which will be described throughout the chapter:

- Include family members and other caregivers in patient education.
- Offer a variety of training opportunities and certifications.
- Integrate health care and research into everyday life.

DOD already does some of these activities in one or more locations. For instance, family members and caregivers can be actively engaged in the rehabilitation process, including attending therapy sessions with their loved one. On the other hand, DOD has a desire to more fully integrate research into rehabilitation.

Summary of Civilian Rehabilitation Site Visitation

Our analysis of civilian centers for specialty rehabilitative care included four sites. We will describe how sites were selected and then discuss the objectives of our site observations. These observations will illustrate the relationships between a center's core values in health care delivery, the patient population they serve, and the structure built into their health care provider teams.

Site Selection

When selecting civilian health care facilities to visit, our team produced a list of candidate facilities based on hospital reputation and ranking ("Best Hospitals," undated). In consultation with EACE leadership, we developed an approved list of programs to contact and schedule for site visits. Of the total of six sites we contacted, the following four sites agreed to host our team:

- The Spaulding Rehabilitation Network, Boston, Massachusetts
- TIRR Memorial Hermann, Houston, Texas
- The Shirley Ryan AbilityLab, Chicago, Illinois
- The Shepherd Center, Atlanta, Georgia

Following correspondence with health care providers and hospital administration, we were invited to tour rehabilitation facilities, treatment rooms, research spaces, and other areas that contribute to the care of patients rehabilitating amputations.

Site Observations

Each site visit took place over the course of one or two days with an assorted mix of facility tours, discussions with health care provider teams, staff interviews, and observations of patient appointments within clinics.

The objective of the site visits was twofold: (1) to determine the site's strengths in terms of rehabilitation services and (2) to understand ways that each site provides care for patients (i.e., silo versus team approach). We took notes during visits and detailed our observations about the organization's goals, the patient populations they serve, and the structure of their health care delivery via their health care providers.

Hospital Focus and Specialization in Rehabilitation

The opening session of our site visits provided an opportunity to learn about the foundational aims and mission of the health care services and facilities provided at each site. While the core values were largely consistent, each site presented a unique emphasis in its overarching goals and operational strategies.

The Spaulding Rehabilitation Network

The Spaulding Rehabilitation Network provides inpatient care out of a new facility overlooking the Charlestown Navy Yard. The inpatient rehabilitation hospital serves a broad network across the greater Boston area and Cape Cod. There are also over 20 outpatient rehabilitation facilities. At the main, inpatient facility, a lot of the patient rooms have views of the water, and access to all treatment areas are adjoined in one location. The health care provider team has experienced unique demands related to patient confidentiality and media requests following the Boston Marathon bombing, and they have carried that learning experience into their new facility. The staff speak very highly of the DOD models for amputee care and seek to provide care for more military service members to further enhance their culture of health care delivery.

The Institute for Rehabilitation and Research Memorial Hermann

TIRR Memorial Hermann provides amputee care with a vetted health care provider network. The vetting process ensures alignment of prosthetics and orthotics companies with the values of the amputee clinic and requires an investment of time in clinic for a mix of health care professionals to be present at all patient appointments. Relationships with the University of Texas Health Sciences Center at Houston Medical School and Baylor College of Medicine provide a strong connection to continuous education, fellowship training opportunities, and dedicated resources for research collaboration. Of note is their ongoing investment in and customization of electronic medical record, which reflect a capability to standardize data collection from patient care with reduced documentation effort. Various members of leadership at TIRR Memorial Hermann have past involvement in military medicine and rehabilitation or current roles in committees for amputee care clinical practice guidelines.

The Shirley Ryan AbilityLab

The Shirley Ryan AbilityLab was a reimagining of the Rehabilitation Institute of Chicago to extend the clinical expertise of care teams as a "clinical engine" behind their research enterprise. Their reimagined care model consists of scientists, engineers, doctors, nurses, patients, and therapists working together in an immersive way with the focus and purpose of care being on asking new or different questions. The Shirley Ryan AbilityLab turns training gyms into ability labs with floors specific to thinking and speaking, legs and walking, arms and hands, and strength and endurance, and pediatric and patient rooms into innovation centers (with floors dedicated to brain cancer and other diseases and ailments).

The Shepherd Center

The Shepherd Center is a post-acute rehabilitation facility built around model systems (i.e., spinal cord injury and acquired brain injury) for patients with long-term health care needs. It has an extensive community of donors, and many services and features of their health care delivery model are built around the engagement of patient families and support networks. In addition, the Shepherd Center is home to the largest recreation technology program in the United States (Shepherd Center, undated-d) and supports multiple U.S. paralympic athletes.

Patient Population Types and Volume Served

Our four sites have all provided amputee care in traumatic cases. However, the areas served and their affiliate network for patient referrals led to some variety in the patient populations treated. These client demographics further demonstrate how each site provides a unique emphasis to their health care delivery models.

The Spaulding Rehabilitation Network

The patient population for amputee care is often 60–70-year-old male patients associated with oncology, high-level amputation, or disarticulation, while a portion of cases includes some traumatic injury involving burns, snowmobile accidents, and other outdoor injuries. Complex medical cases due to sepsis infection have been treated. Inpatient referrals come through the referral network; patients stay for approximately 13 days, with roughly 10 percent returning for prosthetic training and a boot camp program. Currently, the Spaulding Rehabilitation Hospital has 4,000 inpatient admissions annually and 140,000 annual outpatient visits (Spaulding Rehabilitation Network [SRN], undated-b). Following the Boston Marathon bombing, Spaulding provided care for 32 victims, including 15 amputees (SRN, undated-a).

The Institute for Rehabilitation and Research Memorial Hermann

The amputee patient population for TIRR Memorial Hermann is far-reaching and diverse, and its services are targeted to international patients, Spanish-speaking patients, line workers from electric companies, construction workers, and oil and gas industry workers. A special patient subgroup of women includes cases of quadruple amputation due to sepsis infection. Patient volumes across inpatient and outpatient programs are reflected in the specialty rehabilitation practice (i.e., neurologic, orthopaedic, and general rehabilitation) on the order of 150 patients annually (TIRR Memorial Hermann, undated-a). The percentage of patients with amputations is less than 30 percent of the specialty rehabilitation population.

The Shirley Ryan AbilityLab

A new facility for the Shirley Ryan AbilityLab has increased capacity for rehabilitation to 210 beds with a maximum capacity for 360 in downtown Chicago. Additional sites support regional coverage and have an average of 20–30 years of operations; there are

29 sites altogether (six inpatient facilities, 17 outpatient facilities, and eight day-rehabilitation facilities), which provide 194 beds. Patients receiving care at the Shirley Ryan AbilityLab from beyond the regional area are referred via Global Services. The Global Services coordination team addresses the needs and treatment coordination for international and TRICARE patients. Another patient population noted was bariatric patients. During clinical observation, it was noted that most patients served are not likely to return to work or have already retired. With in-house prosthetics and orthotics capabilities, the Shirley Ryan AbilityLab has limb loss and impairment service as a core component of its health care delivery model (Shirley Ryan AbilityLab [SRAL], undated-c).

The Shepherd Center

Amputee patients at the Shepherd Center typically arrive as outpatients, typically between three to 33 days post injury. Amputee patients fall under the care practices of the Shepherd Center's model systems, including spinal cord injury, brain injury, multiple sclerosis, spine and chronic pain, and other neuromuscular conditions. With a history of service spanning more than four decades, the Shepherd Center has grown to a 152-bed hospital that treats more than 900 inpatients, 575 day-program patients, and more than 7,100 outpatients each year (Shepherd Center, undated-a).

Health Care Provider Team Structures for Amputee Care

The differences in patient populations and caseloads have produced a variety of staffing strategies and partnerships for continuous coverage of patient treatment services. The following patient scheduling strategies and health care provider teams were observed during our visit to civilian sites for rehabilitation.

The Spaulding Rehabilitation Network

The health care provider team includes case managers, occupational therapists and PTs, plus social workers by consult. While Spaulding does not have in-house prosthetists, there are community-based prosthetists present during Wednesday clinics. A special interest group for amputee prosthetics holds monthly calls for training and discussions. There has been discussion to create a one-stop facility for integrated health care delivery, and much credit is given to the DOD standards of care for changes toward consolidation of health care delivery.

The Institute for Rehabilitation and Research Memorial Hermann

The staffing model of outpatient clinics utilizes thematic days for scheduling of patients by status (new versus returning) and need (lower versus upper extremity prosthesis). With the support of outside prosthetic companies, this model allowed for a prosthetist to be in the room with the physical medicine and rehabilitation doctor, a nurse, and any case manager(s) or caregivers supporting the patient. Additional services such as PT or counseling are supported from the same site by appointment, but the psychologist support is not full time.

The Shirley Ryan AbilityLab

The health care delivery team includes a host of providers and trainees. Along with the physical medicine and rehabilitation doctor, there were two fellows in training at the time of our visit. In-house prosthetists are also on hand with an additional trainee in prosthetics. One patient (funded by workman's compensation) came with a case manager and was matched with an additional case manager for the Shirley Ryan Ability-Lab. There is also a nurse to capture notes prior to and during the doctor's assessment. Patient tracking technologies facilitate care-on-the-move so that medications or less intrusive medical tasks can be administered within the AbilityLab spaces instead of holding patients still in the innovation centers. Freedom of movement for the patients maximizes their access and participation in functional rehabilitation.

In other areas of the hospital, the AbilityLab design of space and infrastructure is highly modular and customizable to support of patients and providers. The custom features allow for creativity in rehabilitation treatment, but also provide opportunities for researchers to continuously review prospective clinical practice guidelines. In addition to including features that allow for protections to staff and patients (e.g., an overhead weight-bearing support system above an irregular sequence of stairs between floors provides safety for patients relearning to walk), there are dedicated spaces for researchers to conduct studies just beyond the view of patients.

The Shepherd Center

The health care provider teams are led by physicians, and all providers are employed by the Shepherd Center. Each service team is composed of a nurse practitioner, case manager, occupational therapist, PT, recreational therapist, speech and language pathologist, and psychologist (for neurological and brain service). Many of the case managers have a background in social work. By consult, a chaplain and plastic surgery are available to the physician-led service teams. This team-based care model strengthens the interaction across providers. Also of note is that the physician's grand rounds take place in the gym.

Teaming during intake and provision of care is another aspect of the staffing structure at the Shepherd Center. The documentation of core competencies for amputee care is broad and used as part of the staffing and care practices. A culture of serving with the patient's best interest in mind allows for fixed team structures to get access to specialty experience with amputee care across staff and then refer out if the treatment options in house no longer continue to make progress toward patient goals. The health care provider network can refer to a network of community services and expertise outside of Shepherd based on specific patient needs.

Strategies for Building Core Competencies in Amputee Care

The key concerns and challenges we observed among civilian health care providers did not represent areas where they were unable to provide care. In fact, these concerns simply highlighted the complexities of amputation rehabilitation that the sites were actively engaging to address by building competencies that elevate patient health outcomes and quality of life.

In this section, we will summarize our understanding of the best practices across the centers we visited, particularly those that may be of interest to DOD centers of excellence in traumatic injury and amputation rehabilitation. While some practices are similar to those presented earlier in this chapter, others are a result of explicit decisions that the civilian sites made in order to improve patient outcomes.

Given that reimbursement is an issue for civilian rehabilitation providers but not for DOD providers, we do not discuss it in detail.

Health Care Provider Workforce Pipeline and Training

A key consideration is the cultivation of civilian health care provider teams for competency in amputation rehabilitation. In conversations with providers in the civilian care setting, some raised concerns across the spectrum of recruitment, training (or experience), and retention.

Lessons Learned from Experience in Amputation Rehabilitation

Most health care providers shared how their formal training involved very little preparation for handling the needs of patients who have experienced a traumatic amputation. Providers must have the passion to serve patients with chronic needs and/or disabilities. With other patients, it is possible for compensation to be better and the ultimate outcomes to be more rewarding at the point of patient discharge (e.g., final level of restoration and functional ability). Furthermore, there may be a higher challenge to entry for health care providers who are fundamentally less comfortable with the level or degree of injury associated with traumatic events or chronic diseases underlying a medical decision for amputation.

Training for health care providers is a critical issue given the highly specialized area of traumatic care in civilian patient populations with amputations. A provider's first-time experience with providing amputation rehabilitation introduces multiple challenges beyond internalization of the terms and fundamental techniques in the standard of care. These challenges include looking at or touching the limb, facing patient grief and despondency, and protecting wounds at the prosthetic training phase, among others.

Retention strategies must contend with the natural concerns of career progression in addition to various threats to burnout and resignation among health care providers. Burnout is a risk when the time available to find solutions to unique patient needs interferes with personal time away from the hospital. In addition, the variability of patient or family member responsiveness to the treatment plan can increase the strain of delivering a standard of care. Where one patient may make no effort to work with the provider team, another may express dissatisfaction with the rate of progress toward more aggressively set personal goals for functional ability. When considering staffing needs in the face of turnover, or when skill degradation begins to occur because providers are not treating enough patients with complex wounds such as those resulting from a traumatic amputation, management must appropriately invest in training opportunities to cultivate deeper experiences and core competencies. The intense exposure to emotional experiences working with this patient population is likely unique—because of the significant loss amputation patients have experienced, the complex nature of their cases, often with co-occurring conditions, and the long recovery process—and can result in higher than normal turnover rates if not acknowledged and addressed.

Best Practices for Department of Defense Consideration: Hire and Train Passionate, Adaptive Employees

Civilian health care facilities expressed that patient needs are best served when the staff working with them have a passion for the treatment of chronic health needs and disability. This requires selective hiring techniques, possibly targeting job seekers with experience working with these patients or hiring from educational programs that offer training in amputation rehabilitation. This patient population, and each individual patient, has unique needs, as well as unique responses to the intense treatment and rehabilitation required to meet functional goals. They face setbacks and may at times feel discouraged; this is when flexibility and a diverse toolkit become important provider assets. Hiring, encouraging, and supporting provider adaptability and creativity is a best practice. One civilian rehabilitation center provider spoke of wandering the aisles of discount stores looking for items that could be repurposed to help a patient accomplish small day-to-day tasks. When considering the stressors of the work environment, two of the civilian sites discussed their involvement in the Schwartz Seminar, which allows health care providers to share the difficulties of providing care during periods of high emotional duress and the stress of making decisions laden with ethical considerations. The ability to heal others while sustaining oneself is critical to the retention of health care providers in the field. Strategies for combatting "compassion fatigue" are valuable to ensure that health care providers build trust with their patients and manage tactful dialogues on goal-setting and commitment to a plan of rehabilitation.

Balancing Patient Treatment Risks and Benefits: Post-Surgical to Post-Acute Phases

A challenge during rehabilitation is tracking the risk-to-benefit ratio for individual patients, where benefits are measured as gains in function, strength, and mobility, and risks include falls, injury, or other physical, emotional, and safety issues that can occur as the patient works through increasingly difficult steps in rehabilitation. The balance between risk and benefit changes according to post-injury patient time engaging with the health care system.

Lessons Learned from Experience in Amputation Rehabilitation

Beginning in the hospital setting, there is a need to optimize the set of solutions targeting activities of daily living. For instance, when one technology or strategy is introduced or taught, how does it influence the options down the road in dealing with other fundamental activities in life? The best practices observed sought to minimize the time and distance of communications across the health care providers (e.g., having all present during patient visit to clinic). Another strategy is to ensure that a provider who has cared for a similar patient case in the past is consulted or teamed with the service of new patients. In terms of rehabilitation and therapy, there is a strong emphasis on getting patients ready for activity as soon as it is safe to begin. The safety concerns for supporting patients have been met with many high-tech solutions to reduce the risk of falls or injury, and such equipment is in high demand due to the limited resources to procure, operate, and maintain it. By creating a modular rehabilitation plan, some facilities have allowed for greater flexibility in giving patients a choice of activities, while also sustaining the availability of specialized staff members involved in the therapy practice. In addition to the modular plan, another strategy involves blocking out access times for different patient groups, as well as cross-training therapists on the proper use of equipment.

For outpatients learning to reintegrate in society, wheelchairs are a necessary stepping stone en route to independent walking with a prosthesis unless a wheelchair itself is the final goal for mobility. When a new or revised prosthesis is obtained, the old solution is not given away or thrown out. The old prosthetic, like a wheelchair, will be retained by the patient as a spare tool placed within inventory for resiliency should the new one break or not achieve a suitable fit. Expert health care providers seek to match the type of technology, in terms of sophistication, cost, and complexity, with the patient's level of training and comfort to progress with independent mobility. Best practices are not clearly specified in this regard, as the providers must justify medical necessity for all core technologies and each add-on component or feature. An understanding of patients' funding sources and constraints is equally as important as an awareness of their level of training and comfort to progress with mobility goals.

All patients who experience amputation are prospective candidates for newer treatment procedures and technologies as they emerge. However, any new treatment (e.g., pharmaceutic, therapeutic, or technological) comes with a cycle of integration to the patient's lifestyle: (1) familiarization/interest, (2) fitting, and (3) normalization. Failure during the cycle means falling back to a solution within the patient's inventory of spare tools. Success in the cycle does not come without the burden and effort of going through the cycle again. A new technology or treatment is not reason enough to justify repetition of the journey. This challenge is one that noninvasive, emerging technologies must address. In the world of high-tech prostheses, we observed that machine learning in computerized prosthetics has shown some benefits during trials following a familiarization and training period. Also, pattern mapping of other electromyography (EMG) signals is a technology that seeks to map dynamic controls of prosthetics (i.e., robotic arms) to different muscle groups (i.e., chest muscles). Surgically involved treatments include an added challenge for patients, who must undergo a healing phase in advance of the cycle of integration. Osseointegration, a bone-fused prosthesis, has been discussed as a procedure to limit or reduce the issues of skin integrity and fit of prosthesis at the socket (St.-Jean and Fish, 2011). Alternatively, targeted muscle rein-nervation (TMR) is a surgical process to reposition nerve endings into new muscles to retain the residual firing signal within alternative muscle groups (Cheesborough et al., 2015). The procedure has benefits if paired with pattern mapping, but it has now been associated with some potential for enhanced pain management and prevention of neuromas. The benefits, if validated, are enormous, given that the cycle of integra-tion is a considerable burden to the patient. For some older patients, surgical revision is simply too risky.

Best Practices for Department of Defense Consideration: Include Family Member and Other Caregivers in Patient Education

The best approach to increase informed decisionmaking is to include all stakeholders in health care education. Patients must make many decisions during their rehabilita-tion, but the supporting role that family members or caregivers play can better inform the risk-benefit balance.

Creating a shared space for patient education can promote family engagement with challenging treatment decisions and even ways to better express and communi-cate common needs and discomforts. These feelings must be presented by patients to their health care provider, but they must also be understood by the family and friends who are most accessible after discharge. With physical and online resources to support the discovery and description of common challenges that patients will face, there is a better likelihood of having patients advocating for their best interests. The Henry B. Betts LIFE Center at the Shirley Ryan AbilityLab provides resources and staff to assist patients, families, and health professionals in their search for health information (SRAL, undated-b). Under the circumstances, health care providers will also have a better understanding of patient needs and how to manage their long-term health care.

Coordinated Support of Health Care Providers with Amputation Rehabilitation Expertise

Health care providers bring specialized skills to patients with the aim of healing and restoration. The dynamic and complex nature of people's needs can bring providers to the limits of what they can offer, but the emotional reactions by patients and their family can amplify frustrations with the scope of options at hand. These are some of the best practices at work to maintain an experienced and fulfilled roster of health care providers.

Lessons Learned from Experience in Amputation Rehabilitation

The coordination of provider teams and physician service teams requires active review and forecasting to ensure the match of skills to patient needs in a hospital. Concerns about core competency and readiness to provide care were expressed at multiple sites experiencing staff turnover (i.e., nursing shortage) and inability to expand services (i.e., to attract providers to this specialty care field). In response, the Shepherd Center has a mentoring program for the first three months. All sites invest in conferences, workshops, and seminars for training. Technique can be practiced on mock-patients (i.e., dummies) or model patients (i.e., prior patients with amputations). For emerging topics and research awareness, civilian sites create relationships with local institutions for health care education for physicians, therapists, counselors, and prosthetists. Some efforts have also been made to hire dual-hatted clinicians who conduct research but maintain a clinical practice two to three days a week.

The "champions" of health care quality at any facility are those who have taken ownership of the standard of care and advancement of excellence. One best practice demonstrated across civilian rehabilitation centers relates to the internal capacity to fund early-stage, investigative research. Such research can validate provider-initiated efforts to formalize new techniques and strategies for providing care, while the collections of data on patient outcomes builds a base of evidence for other practitioners to consider. These opportunities can be used as incentives based on merit or tenure, but the capacity to conduct this form of research sends a signal to reinforce how individual contributions to fulfill the mission of quality care are desired and rewarded. The bricks construct the building, but the people build the institution.

Best Practices for Department of Defense Consideration: Offer a Variety of Training Opportunities and Certifications

Options to maintain competency and expertise in amputation rehabilitation include just-in-time training on top of foundational skills or coordinated support of specific skills. Moreover, just-in-time training can be amplified by incorporating patient models and certifying the health care provider team's training in rehabilitation.

Patient models offer a real-world context during training in ways that go beyond the core mechanics of performing health care activities. These activities take place amid challenging emotions and include the potential for noncompliance by patients. In addition, the realism added by using patient models allows for repeated practice of health care activities including assessing skin temperature, pain, and limb movement. Exposure to patient models is a valuable complement to complement simulated exercises and other resources. Peer counselors and mentors participants can be a strong partner in this regard.

Mandatory training in rehabilitation for all staff members is a foundational effort that goes hand in hand with specialized training opportunities. TIRR Memorial Hermann specifically stated that patient outcomes improved after mandating that all nurses become certified rehabilitation registered nurses (CRRN). Expertise in this special area of practice is documented through the certification, which is also approved by the VA (Association of Rehabilitation Nurses, undated). This effort is in place at the Shirley Ryan AbilityLab and Shepherd Center as well.

Focusing on Foundational Skills to Prepare Patients for Their Journey to Recovery

Across all civilian rehabilitation health care facilities, it was clear that there is only a limited amount of time for health care delivery and patient healing. The comments from providers everywhere indicated that the optimal solution does not always get figured out during their shift. Patients are not expected to come to grips with their new realities in life in just two weeks until discharge. For these reasons, patient treatment and education is best offered with an eye toward how patients can leverage their resources of support to heal and advocate for themselves without limitation on time spent with a health care provider. Civilian health care facilities have created techniques and infrastructure to better support opportunities for relationship building within families and communities.

Lessons Learned from Experience in Amputation Rehabilitation

The most effective way for patients to understand how life will change and to learn how to adapt after discharge is by simulating the activities of daily living. Most facilities have spaces that replicate the home setting to integrate goals at home with the therapy sessions and plan for rehabilitation. A best practice in this regard is the provision of housing support to families of patients adjacent to the health care facility. This allows family members to witness the progression of rehabilitation and practice activities of daily living with their loved one in a protective environment before taking on full responsibilities at home. The creation of family spaces is another means to support. Such spaces allow the family to take time to grieve at their own pace, with some privacy, during therapy sessions and transition points through the day.

Communication of needs and emotions is a challenge for patients as they struggle to understand the full scope of changes to their lives. Peer counseling programs are a clear best practice in assisting patients with communication and coping strategies for their grief. Whether the need is to raise an issue with health care providers or better explain needs to family members, peer counselors can serve families as experienced guides to restructuring day-to-day activities in life. Some models include training and certification of peer counselors for a matching process (i.e., the Shirley Ryan Ability-Lab Peer Mentor Program [SRAL, 2018]); others use referrals to outside organizations with their own program offering (e.g., 22Kill [22Kill, undated]). The benefits from these relationships can be further tuned toward topics of safety and advocacy as patients rebound from periods of grief and frustration. Peer counseling can help patients advocate for themselves by guiding patients to resources or the right questions to ask, learning how to safely try new things, and understanding what will remain unknown or part of the discovery process. Safety benefits can begin immediately by learning how to communicate concerns to caregivers or the health care provider team, while long-term benefits can come from knowledge about future red flags to watch for in terms of health maintenance.

Regaining a sense of belonging or purpose is fundamental to the multilayered challenges for amputation rehabilitation. Opportunities for joint training and education are linked to health care through recreational therapy. The best practices in this regard involve efforts to provide adaptive gym and therapy spaces with sporting activities that expose patients to healthy competition and teamwork. The network of recreational therapy programs is highly driven by donor funding and volunteer staff. Training and standards are transferred by word of mouth and peer mentoring. Despite the challenges and lack of resources, the outcomes of these programs directly target the patient's self-image. Coordinators of such programs are repeatedly told about moments when participants said, "I never thought I would do that again" or "I felt like I'm on a team again." Those realizations and feelings were expressions from military veterans in mixed company with civilians, and the ability to have those feelings are tightly linked to the identity of a military service member within their unit.

Best Practices for Department of Defense Consideration: Integrate Health Care and Research into Daily Activities

Civilian health care facilities for rehabilitation apply varied strategies to merge health care activities and safety measures with everyday life. An active lifestyle comes with greater integration with local services and exploration of resources or strategies that have shown success for others with amputations. Two scenarios suggest how the DOD can further enhance amputation rehabilitation for military service members in ways that are not currently standardized across DOD settings.

The first concerns the design and support of inclusive environments. For instance, adaptive gyms and stores can serve to ease transition back into the community. Adaptive gyms have been established for people with disabilities, including those with amputations, while also providing monthly memberships to able-bodied customers. This form of integration allows for specialty equipment to be procured and maintained within a revenue-generating organization. While donations can be collected for high-priced items, the revenue can pay for staff salaries and facilities operating costs. At the same time, the community would witness those with amputations achieving goals beyond the rehabilitation phase. The Shirley Ryan AbilityLab operates a fitness center (SRAL, undated-a) for people of all abilities, while the Shepherd Center runs Beyond Therapy (Shepherd Center, undated-b) as a self-paid, activity-based therapy program.

The second involves structuring research into health care practice with a niche population of patients. The streamlined integration of research into daily operations helps to build the evidence base for patient-centered goals. For example, tracking data on post-acute treatment can help to indicate the values and impact of in-hospital treatment strategies. In turn, adjustments to in-hospital treatment strategies can promote more successful post-acute outcomes for a greater percentage of the patients served. The Shirley Ryan AbilityLab boasts the creation of in-clinic (AbilityLab) spaces for researchers and customizable equipment (i.e., benches and patient lifts) to facilitate reconfiguration and quantification of novel treatment protocols for optimized outcomes. The Shepherd Center demonstrated that alternative data collection protocols can be trialed and demonstrated through outpatient programs (e.g., SHARE Military Initiative) (Shepherd Center, undated-c) to better inform and revise hospital-based data collection protocols. With the goal of having providers spend more time treating than documenting, the national database from TBI model systems sites (TIRR Memorial Hermann, undated-b) represents a high value for documenting standard of care with validity across health care delivery models and geography. Similar efforts could support the evidence base underlying patient-centered care strategies across sites providing amputation rehabilitation.

CHAPTER FIVE

Conclusions and Recommendations

The ultimate aim of our study was to identify and document core competencies that health care providers in nine service areas need to have when providing rehabilitative services to service members who experienced deployment-related amputations. With the number of patients with new deployment-related amputations entering DOD's rehabilitation program decreasing during much of the last decade, this study addresses an important, widening gap by documenting competency information now, before knowledge about what is needed to provide high-quality rehabilitation services to those with amputations is forgotten. Examining competencies at the present time also allows for a determination of the skills that are at the most risk of atrophy given the decline in patient volume.

Methods and Findings

We conducted and analyzed approximately 110 interviews with patients and family members, health care providers, and subject matter experts about which services are integral for optimal rehabilitation, areas where skill atrophy might occur in a low patient volume environment, and best practices and behaviors observed in military treatment facilities where amputation rehabilitation occurs. Using the findings from those interviews, existing competency frameworks and/or practice standards, and information from the *Care of the Combat Amputee* (Lenhart, Pasquina, and Cooper, 2009), we proposed a set of competencies that were common to the nine types of services for which we were able to develop competencies: behavioral health, case management, diet/nutrition, occupational therapy, orthopaedic surgery, PT, physical medicine and rehabilitation, prosthetics and orthotics, and biomedical engineering. For each service, we also proposed a set of behaviors. We then conducted a two-wave TES in which experts in each field had an opportunity to provide feedback on the proposed competencies and behaviors, as well as rate them for their importance and frequency in amputation rehabilitation. The final set of competencies that emerged from that process includes: (1) teamwork, (2) patient and family education, (3) military and other cultural awareness, (4) patient-centered care, (5) evidence-based practice, and (6) ethical and professional behavior. A complete set of behaviors for each service is included in Appendix E.

Limitations

Our study has some limitations worth acknowledging. First, we conducted the study several years after the height of recent wars. This meant that our interviews covered a smaller subset of the provider population (overall and with experience with this patient population) than if this study had been conducted earlier. The information we obtained from interviews and TESs was valuable yet we might have had more respondents with different experiences if data collection occurred during a different time period. Given that memories fade over time, it is possible that respondents provided us with the most salient critical behaviors that they remembered and that nuanced behaviors were forgotten and not reported to us.

We also identified other services and disciplines that are integral to amputation rehabilitation but for which we were unable to define competencies. For instance, we were unable to identify enough recreational therapists and dermatologists (or wound management providers more generally) to meet the minimum requirements established in our administrative approvals. It is possible that the same six competencies apply to these providers in the DOD setting, but we were unable to validate that and did not develop behaviors for these types of services. The feedback they provided during the interviews that we were able to conduct still benefited our analysis.

The findings from our interviews were weighted toward administrative planning and organization design issues and were lighter on clinical care. We assumed providers had the appropriate medical background, although we acknowledge that those skills may atrophy without enough exposure to the right patient mix. Complementary to the results of this analysis are findings on care delivery, particularly the literature on health care provided at WRAMC.

The TESs had several limitations. We would ideally have convened technical expert panels for each of the services, which would have allowed us to discuss each behavior in real time. However, due to the length of the surveys and constraints on provider time, we were unable to bring providers together in such meetings. However, using an asynchronous, modified Delphi-like approach also has a number of advantages, as it allows all participants an equal opportunity to participate and to be more candid in their feedback due to the anonymous nature of the surveys, as well as overcoming constraints related to geography and scheduling (Janke et al., 2016; Yousuf, 2007).

Another limitation was the number of respondents for each survey. We had between four and eight participants in each round one survey. Those experts who responded may be especially invested in quality improvement efforts related to amputation rehabilitation, and therefore may not be representative of the larger population of providers from a given discipline. That said, all experts were invited based on their experience with this population, and therefore were especially well situated to provide feedback about these competencies and behaviors. In addition, because we focused on behaviors for which there was consensus across services, we have greater confidence that our results do not simply reflect the perceptions or attitudes of a single service area.

Additionally, it is important to note that the behaviors identified within each competency across services are intended to be *representative* of each competency. This means that the behavior lists are not exhaustive. Therefore, there are almost certainly additional critical behaviors within each competency for each service, and there is room to expand upon this effort. A related issue is that within each competency across services, there was a number of behaviors for which consensus was not achieved (i.e., the low-agreement behaviors). Unfortunately, it was beyond the scope of this study to further explore the reasons why consensus was not achieved for these behaviors. It may be that these behaviors are simply not representative of a given competency. However, it may also be that there are external factors that contribute to within-discipline differences—for example, there may be differences in practice by treatment setting (e.g., inpatient versus outpatient) or based on the structure of a multidisciplinary team (e.g., which role is assigned to which provider on a given team). Future investigations could explore the factors that contributed to the lack of agreement on these behaviors.

Finally, our charge was to document the competencies needed by providers who rehabilitate service members and veterans who have experienced deployment-related amputation(s), and our primary source of information was interviews we conducted with DOD providers. In doing so, we made the assumption that the knowledge, skills, and abilities that these providers have is what should be documented and built upon. We did not explicitly evaluate the care that DOD provided to this patient population. We did summarize some of the literature on patient outcomes, including functional restoration, quality of life, and return to duty rates among patients with amputation, but those studies were not specifically about outcomes following care delivered by DOD. As we describe below, as DOD develops metrics to measure skill levels and assess competencies and behaviors, it will be important to link those metrics to patient outcomes, arguably the most important measure in evaluating quality of care.

We now turn to recommendations on how EACE, the MHS, and individual providers ought to use this information going forward.

Recommendations

Our first recommendation concerns next steps that need to occur to officially validate and formalize these competencies in military settings. As a reminder, our TESs served only as an initial validation of our competencies. We included experts outside of the setting for which the competencies were developed, and we did not explicitly tie competencies and behaviors to performance or level of expertise. Some of our recommendations pertain to further validating the findings from this research. Without formalization, there is little chance of the competencies we identified being accepted within these settings.

Recommendation 1: Core Competencies Need to Be Formally Accepted by Those Leading and Working in Military Health Care Settings

For any new process to be effective, it is important that stakeholders who are being asked to use it to provide feedback. Murray et al. (2010), using normalization process theory, noted several key questions that must be answered before new processes/interventions (i.e., use of a new competency framework) have a chance of being successful. These questions focus on four main areas—coherence, cognitive participation, collective action, and reflexive monitoring—and are posited as necessary to maximize the chance for a successful intervention. Examples of questions that need to be asked before interventions are implemented include whether those being asked to use the intervention understand the purpose of the intervention (coherence), think the intervention is a good idea (cognitive participation), view work being affected in a positive way (collective action), and perceive the intervention as advantageous to providers and/or patients (reflexive monitoring).

Adapting Murray et al.'s (2010) approach and having EACE or another entity champion the importance of the competency framework within MTFs will help in the messaging of this framework as it is implemented. Further, socializing these core competencies among leaders, administrators, and providers at MTFs provides the opportunity to obtain buy-in from providers and leaders/administrators. Buy-in can help lead to (1) the competency framework becoming part of the standard operating procedures initially and part of the broader culture eventually and (2) common understanding/agreement about how competencies should be used in these settings. Part of the buy-in process involves allowing providers to add additional behaviors relevant to the core competencies; our behaviors are examples and not inclusive of all behaviors one would need to demonstrate for any one competency. It is important to note that we sought the participation of both DOD and civilian experts for the TESs for this study in order to have large enough sample sizes, as well as to leverage the expertise of providers who work outside of the DOD setting. According to DOD, validation of competencies would be done by a representative sample or census of the current workforce for whom the competencies apply.[1] Seeking buy-in and input from DOD providers on the competencies we developed will further validate them.

This recommendation is focused on socialization within military health care settings yet we acknowledge that there are other military entities that also need to buy

---

[1]   DODI 1400.25, Vol. 250, 2016.

into the proposed competency framework, likely before the military health care settings are approached. Examples of these entities that might help legitimize the competency framework include MEDCOM, the DHA, and the DHB.

Recommendation 2: Once Competencies Are Accepted, Those in Military Health Care Settings Must Decide How to Use Them

As noted previously, competency modeling yields competencies that provide an organizing framework for behaviors that one needs to perform for a given job. As a result, competencies can be used in multiple ways—when making hiring decisions, appraising performance, identifying training needs, and so on—and ideally competencies will represent a foundation upon which these multiple uses are oriented. We provide an example of how competencies can be used for performance appraisal purposes.

In early 2000s, MEDCOM developed and posted competency assessments/tools for many health care provider positions on the Tri-Service Healthcare Competency Assessment website (The Military Health System, undated). These competency tools are used to document six types of information about personnel and as a result are referred to as six-sided folders, or competency assessment files (CAFs). The information collected in the CAF consists of: (1) background information such as career assignments and skill likes/dislikes, (2) current practice information including job description and evidence of competency assessment, (3) professional education, military training, and other achievements, (4) information about licensure and certification, 5) information about professional experience including letters of reference and/or recognition, and (6) additional relevant information. Given that MEDCOM has already developed the format and recommended way that the CAF should be used, it would be possible to integrate the competencies we identified into the CAF framework.

Recommendation 3: Military Health System Leadership Should Adopt a Proficiency Framework for Assessing Individual and System-Wide Competencies

For example, the NAS, Engineering, and Medicine has developed the Five Levels of Clinical Competence Framework and recommended delineating skill levels for competencies. This delineation allows one to determine what mix of skills is currently in the workforce and what skills are still needed. Table 5.1 contains the five skill levels and the descriptions provided by NAS, along with an amputation-related application for PM&R providers.

RAND Arroyo Center recommends that MHS, EACE, and DHA leadership adopt the NAS clinical competence framework, or a similar framework with a delineation of skill levels, to establish a desired distribution of proficiency that is needed to provide optimal rehabilitative services to patients with amputation and to conduct a baseline assessment of its current staff. While it might be desirable to have a full staff of experts across the range of services provided to this patient population, that is not likely to be feasible both from a financial perspective and because of the natural turn-

Table 5.1
National Academies of Sciences, Engineering, and Medicine's Five Levels of Clinical Competence, Adapted to Amputation Rehabilitation

Skill Level	Description	Rehabilitation-Related Example for PM&R
Novice	The novice has no experience in the environment in which he or she is expected to perform.	Physician has never worked with patients rehabilitating from an amputation.
Advanced Beginner	The advanced beginner demonstrates marginally acceptable performance and has enough experience to note recurrent meaningful situational components.	Physician has had didactic training in pain management but no experience applying it to rehabilitation.
Competent	Competence is achieved when the individual begins to see his or her actions in terms of long-range goals or plans. This individual demonstrates efficiency, coordination, and confidence in his or her actions.	Board-eligible/certified physician, but has only rotated as a resident at a center where they rehabilitated patients with amputation.
Proficient	The proficient individual perceives situations holistically and possesses the experience to understand what to expect in a given situation.	Board-eligible/certified physician, either starting his or her career at a high-volume, highly ranked civilian rehabilitation center that rehabilitates patients recovering from traumatic amputations (i.e., due to automobile accident).
Expert	The expert has an intuitive and deep understanding of the total situation and is able to deliver complex medical care under highly stressful circumstances.	Physician with years of experience at a high-volume, highly ranked civilian rehabilitation center.

SOURCE: National Academies of Sciences, 2016.

over that occurs within the workforce (possibly heightened due to the emotional intensity of working with amputee patients, as discussed in Chapter Four). Perhaps within a given service, one or two experts are needed for the purposes of training more inexperienced providers, advising in particularly complex cases, and retaining institutional knowledge. The desired skill level mix likely depends upon patient volume and patient need, both today and as projected into the future (in the event of future conflicts, for instance). The desired mix also needs to be determined at the system and installations levels.

In addition, in order to determine what new staff or additional training of existing staff is needed, the NAS framework should be used to develop a baseline of the distribution of clinical competencies among current staff. If the current skill level falls below or is otherwise misaligned with the desired distribution, the MHS, EACE, and the DHA will be able to implement a plan for how to close the gap.

Recommendation 4: Metrics and Assessment Time Frames Associated with Competencies Must Be Validated for Military Health Care Settings

Once a baseline has been established for the current skill mix among providers who rehabilitate patients with amputation, individual providers and the overall mix of clinical competence should be assessed regularly. Linking competencies and behaviors to performance and skill level is an additional step toward validating the competencies identified in this study. Previous research on competencies provides guidance for possible metrics and time frames for assessing competencies. Given the information we documented in this study, one could assess the competencies and associated behaviors (see Appendix E) using a variety of approaches. For example, competencies can be assessed during performance appraisals (which represent one possible use of this framework) by (1) having providers share examples of ways they demonstrate the behaviors in practice, (2) having providers demonstrate the behaviors in simulation exercises, (3) having peers share examples of providers demonstrating these competencies, and (4) having patients provide input about the quality/quantity of these behaviors. The first two approaches are consistent with the version of the CAF approach, in which providers complete a self-assessment of their performance or demonstrate the behavior in a class or in front of an assessor. We also include peers and patients as sources of information because three of the competencies have implications for peers and patients—teamwork, patient and family education, and patient-centered care. In addition, as we discussed in Chapter One and learned during our civilian rehabilitation center site visits described in Chapter Four, patient outcomes are one way to assess the quality of care that is delivered. For this patient population, such outcomes include functional restoration, quality of life, and return to duty rates, although as we noted in Chapter One, what is known about these outcomes is not specific to care provided by DOD, but rather concerns OEF/OIF veterans more generally. Linking metrics to patient outcomes and conducting assessments in such a way that patient outcomes are a focus, especially by including patients and family members in those assessments, will yield improvements in the quality of care.

Once agreement has been reached on how providers will be assessed, MHS leadership needs to be responsible for making sure that there is a clear process regarding which behaviors need to be validated by a supervisor (as is currently outlined in the CAF) and which cannot be validated. For example, one might want to encourage patients to speak up about the patient-centered behaviors and in so doing might solicit anonymous comments, but these would be difficult to validate. In that case, a broader discussion about ways the performance appraisal should be used needs to occur for all stakeholders. For example, would it be wise to make promotion decisions based on patient comments that cannot be corroborated or validated? There are also more distal measures of competence that one might want to consider, such as patient success in rehabilitation or patient/family satisfaction with provider services. Given the team-based approach to rehabilitation, care must be taken when developing a provider-specific metric such as patient success to ensure that the metric reflects the provider of interest and not the team. Alternatively, if a team-based metric is desired, one must determine how team-based metrics fit into individual-level competency assessments. In addition, a time frame for conducting assessments consistent with institutional standards needs to be established. Kak, Burkhalter, and Cooper (2001, p. 5) recommended that "all staff should be assessed prior to employment, during the orientation period, and at least annually thereafter."

Recommendation 5: Once Optimal Skill Mix Has Been Identified, Mitigation Strategies for Competency Gaps Need to Be Developed

Following up on recommendations 3 and 4 will allow leaders in military health care settings to determine what competency gaps exist and how to address these. For example, if leadership assesses the skill distribution among current staff and then finds at the next assessment that distribution has shifted toward a less proficient team of providers, this shift will signal to leadership that additional training or a different approach to hiring is needed. A less proficient staff could be the result of turnover and more junior hires, or it could indicate that the current volume and mix of patients are resulting in an erosion of skills. In either case, adoption of a framework used to empirically measure proficiency allows leadership to address problems as they arise.

If skills are eroding because providers are not working with the right types of patients, partnerships between civilian and military sites might be one way to expose military health care providers to more patients rehabilitating amputations. For example, DOD providers might rotate through a civilian site to care for patients and/or some civilian patients might receive treatment at DOD sites (an example of this is when some Boston Marathon bombing patients received care at WRNMMC [Levine, 2014]). Both approaches require additional approvals—military staff receiving privileges to care for patients at civilian sites for the former; civilian patients receiving congressional approval to receive DOD care in the latter. These types of agreements, which may also take time to establish and be costly, would offer providers an opportunity to gain hands-on experience with, for instance, patients who have traumatic injuries resulting from automobile accidents and who have needs similar to those of young injured service members. Either way, such arrangements offer invaluable opportunities for DOD providers to improve/maintain their skill levels. A second type of partnership is one in which DOD providers serve as educators (for a few days or a full semester) in academic programs, thereby helping to train new students in amputation rehabilitation and relieve some provider shortages (e.g., of physicians [Association of American Medical Colleges, 2018]). Sending DOD providers to education programs would expose entry-level students who might not otherwise learn about this patient population to their needs.[2]

---

[2]   Appendix F provides a brief overview of the exposure to amputation rehabilitation that a few entry-level programs provide.

There are other ways to help providers develop competencies. New hires or staff who have not seen sufficient volume of this patient population may do short rotations through MTFs that rehabilitate relatively more of these patients, such as WRNMMC. EACE sponsors an annual multiday training event called the Federal Advanced Amputation Skills Training (FAAST), which provides attendees with information about best practices in caring for patients who have lost limbs because of combat, injury, or disease. In addition, the State of the Science Symposium brings together researchers and health care providers from a range of rehabilitation centers and programs to share advances and practices for caring for combat amputees. Finally, tools such as clinical practice guidelines and electronic courses are easily accessible to providers at any time for little or no cost.[3]

The best type of training for a given provider depends upon how he or she interacts with a patient and his or her current skill level. For instance, a new hire who is assessed as competent according to the NAS framework likely would not need regular refreshers from online courses but would find value in spending time at Walter Reed when new amputation patients are arriving from an overseas deployment. Due to the nature of their work, surgeons benefit most from hands-on patient experience and may benefit greatly by spending time at a civilian rehabilitation center where they perform surgeries on patients who have experienced a limb injury or amputation from automobile accidents, even if the surgery is different than one performed on a service member with a combat-related amputation.

Finally, there were several lessons learned from our civilian rehabilitation center site visits that may apply to new staff or those whose skills are at risk of atrophying, as we described in the previous two chapters. They include knowledge transfer when an experienced provider is planning to retire or leave; mentoring programs for new staff; consultation between experts and less-experienced staff when a new patient is about to arrive; conferences, workshops, and seminars; mock-patients or model patients; and just-in-time and mandatory training. Whether and which training tools are used at a given health care facility depends upon the specific needs of providers and the patients currently being rehabilitated there.

Conclusion

Following a decade of war and significant investment by DOD to provide state-of-the-art care to service members who experienced deployment-related amputations, this particular patient volume began to decline, and concerns arose regarding how provider

---

[3] One civilian rehabilitation center we visited developed online tools that providers could review when they needed a refresher in a particular clinical technique. These tools or courses can be accompanied by tests that providers take at completion to assess what they learned.

skills could be maintained and sustained during a period of decreased conflict. Our research documented competencies that apply to providers in nine service categories, as well as examples of service category–specific behaviors. Such information is a critical first step toward ensuring DOD can sustain the high quality of care it delivered to patients who experienced amputation(s) since 9/11. We have provided a set of recommendations that serve as a road map for further validating the findings of this study, defining a desired level of proficiency among staff who rehabilitate this patient population, and establishing a plan for routinely assessing the skill mix among providers. Following this guidance will allow DOD to identify any gaps or erosion of skills that arise and to address them through additional training or targeted hiring, while avoiding or minimizing a dip in medical capabilities and experience that has historically occurred during interwar periods.

Context of Battlefield Amputations

An amputation has been, and continues to be, the most visible consequence of warfare, and it is often highlighted by veteran service organizations.[1] Nevertheless, the loss of a limb—a major amputation—is now relatively rare compared to previous wars in terms of the number of these types of injuries, while the percentage of surviving wounded is similar to that of the twentieth century, as shown in Table 2.1.

Since the beginning of combat in 2001, more than 1.3 million Army soldiers have been deployed to Afghanistan and Iraq. Army casualties have numbered over 3,900 "hostile deaths," and over 36,000 "wounded in action" (Defense Casualty Analysis System, 2017), compared with 1,098 major limb amputations and 179 minor limb amputations.[2]

Military wounds, their treatment, and amputations were very different from what had been seen in civilian hospitals. In particular, the number of multi-limb amputations (see Figure A.1) is an indication of the severity of wounds sustained from IEDs and the challenges faced in rehabilitation.

Among those who experienced an amputation, 39 percent of those whose injury happened in OEF lost more than one limb, and among those in OEF and OND, 24 percent were multi-limb, rates that were much higher than the 2–20 percent multiple-

---

[1] A qualitative content analysis of 15 veteran-relevant health content areas/domains on 34 veterans service organizations (VSOs) websites showed that of a "total of 277 health topics . . . the top five . . . [were] insurance/TRICARE/Veterans Administration issues (28.2%), posttraumatic stress disorder (PTSD; 15.5%), disability/amputation/wounds (13.4%), Agent Orange (10.5%), and traumatic brain injury (9.0%)" (Poston et al., 2013, p. 88).

[2] As of February 1, 2016, as reported in Carino (2016a). Major limbs include legs, arms, full hands, and feet. Minor limbs include fingers and toes. Note that the numbers reported do not include "limb salvage" as limb salvage is performed in order to give patients an alternative to amputation. Previously, the Army reported 42 limb salvage procedures as amputations (Carino, 2016b). The choice between limb salvage and amputation of the severely traumatized lower limb is a rather modern concept, as noted in Sanders and Helfet (2004):

> In trauma cases, improved methods of fracture fixation and vessel and nerve repair, along with the selective use of vascularized distant muscle and skin flaps, have provided many opportunities for limb salvage in cases destined for amputation prior to development of these techniques. This approach to limb salvage involves the skills of several specialists during multiple surgical procedures, often followed by prolonged rehabilitation.

Table A.1
Army Amputation Survivors, Civil War, World Wars I and II, Korean War, Vietnam Conflict, and Recent Operations in Afghanistan and Iraq

Conflict	Extremities Wounded	Individuals Wounded	Surviving Amputees	
			Number	Percent of Surviving Wounded
Civil War	Upper	83,536	12,860	15.4
	Lower	89,528	8,002	10.2
	Total	173,064	20,862	12.1
World War I	Upper	55,000	2,359	4.3
	Lower	69,000	2,044	3.0
	Total	154,000	4,378	2.9
World War II	Upper	167,000	3,152	1.9
	Lower	248,000	11,760	4.7
	Total	599,000	14,912	2.5
Korea	Upper	21,002	454	2.2
	Lower	26,270	1,023	3.9
	Total	47,272	1,477	3.1
Vietnam	Total	99,000	5,283	5.3
Afghanistan and Iraq	Major Limb	36,810	1,098	2.9
	Total		1,277	3.4

SOURCES: Beebe and DeBakey, 1952, Table 90, p. 194; Reister, 1975, Table 26, p. 400; Otis and Huntington, 1883, Table 158; Reister, 1973, Table 51, p. 48, Table B-12, p. 160; Author Unknown, 2015; Carino, 2016a, 2016b.

NOTE: The World War II and Korea numbers include nonbattle amputations, which were not included in the World War I numbers. In Korea, there were also 1,120 traumatic amputations as noted in Reznick (2009).

amputee rate reported from World War I, World War II, the Korean War, and the Vietnam War (Krueger, 2012). DOD-wide, from the beginning of hostilities through 2016, there were 1,134 single limb amputations, 463 two-limb amputations, 56 three-limb amputations, and six four-limb amputations. It was reported that the most common cause of injuries leading to an amputation was an explosive device (93 percent). The vast majority (over 80 percent) of the amputations were done the same day as wounding, with 10 percent more than 90 days after the date of injury; these data suggest "that the medical personnel who are initially caring for the injured service members have been consistent in determining which limbs should undergo an acute amputation and those that should undergo an attempted salvage" (Krueger, 2012, p. S442).

Figure A.1
Multi-Limb Amputations: 2001–2016

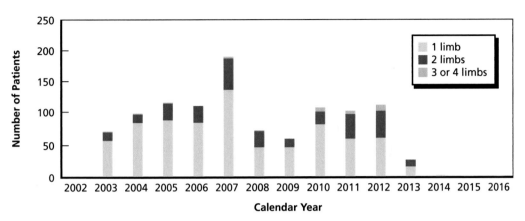

SOURCE: Carino, 2016a.

Studies of Patient Outcomes and Examples of Recent Technological Advancements in Amputation Rehabilitation

In 2010, the VA reported the results of the first national survey of amputees from the Vietnam War and the conflicts in Afghanistan and Iraq, OEF and OIF. The "Survey for Prosthetic Use," conducted in 2007 and 2008, "identified [the] level(s) of limb loss concurrent injuries and illnesses, health status, quality of life, and physical function" (p. vii). In addition, the survey documented service members' "use, replacement, rejection, and abandonment of prosthetic devices and their satisfaction with prosthetic and assistive devices" (Smith and Reiber, 2010, p. vii). The results of the survey clearly showed how much the rehabilitation of amputees had changed in the quarter century that separated Vietnam from OIF/OEF, and the paradigm shift for the DOD and the VA.[1] The result of the paradigm shift is reflected in the way amputees of the two conflicts received their prosthetic, as reported in Table B.1.

After September 11, 2001, DOD initiated "holistic rehabilitation care . . . [at] specialized centers . . . designed to achieve the highest level of physical, psychological, and emotional function in servicemembers with limb loss" (Smith and Reiber, 2010, p. viii). Care from the VA for the Vietnam amputee was clearly less ambitious. Tradi-

Table B.1
Provision of Prosthetic Devices Among Participants in the 2007–2008 Survey for Prosthetic Use Study

Conflict	Percentage Currently Using Prosthetic	Percentage Who Received Prosthetic from Private Source Under Contract with VA	Percentage Who Received Prosthetic from VA	Percentage Who Received Prosthetic from DOD	Percentage Who Received Prosthetic from Multiple Sources
Vietnam	78.2	78.0	16.0	0.9	5.0
OEF/OIF	90.5	42.0	9.0	39.0	10.0

SOURCE: Berke et al., 2010.

---

[1] The term *paradigm shift* is also used to describe the change in Pasquina (2010) and Sigford (2010).

tionally, at the VA all veterans with limb loss "receive[d] prosthetic devices according to their functional level if deemed medically appropriate by their managing physician" (Blough et al., 2010, p. 388). And the VA took "a narrow view of amputation care, focusing only on managing prosthetic devices; . . . the rehabilitation approach was to offer a veteran with a lower-limb loss either a prosthetic device or a wheelchair" (Smith and Reiber, 2010, pp. vii, ix).

To a large extent, the different approach to amputee rehabilitation is a reflection of the different populations served by DOD and the VA. The majority of those with amputations receiving care in VA medical facilities have sustained their amputations because of medical conditions such as diabetes and peripheral vascular disease, and therefore were very different from the new "young, highly trained group of individuals committed to an active lifestyle who are early in their developmental life cycle" (Sigford, 2010, p. xv). Eventually, the VA followed DOD's lead in establishing a program to address the needs of a new group of combat amputees, but not until 2006, and the program was not fully functional until 2010.[2]

The survey results showed greater use of prosthetic devices for OEF/OIF versus Vietnam groups.[3] Satisfaction varied between the two groups depending on the type of amputation,[4] but overall prosthetic satisfaction for those using prostheses was significantly higher in the OIF/OEF cohort than in the Vietnam cohort.[5] However, the rejection rate was higher in the OIF/OEF group than the Vietnam cohort, possibly because

---

[2]   The change was based on the work and recommendations of a task force chartered in 2006. Plans for the new Amputation System of Care were finalized early in 2008, with funding to begin in 2009. The plan included the hiring of new staff and the establishment of Regional Amputation Centers (RACs), and Polytrauma Amputation Network Site (PANS). Amputation Care Team (ACT) and Amputation Points of Contact (APOC) components became fully functional by the end of 2010, as noted in Sigford (2010).

[3]   Specifically, unilateral lower-limb loss was 94 percent for OEF/OIF versus 89 percent for Vietnam; unilateral upper-limb loss utilization rates were 76 percent versus 70 percent, respectively, and utilization rates for multiple limb loss were 92 percent versus 69 percent, respectively, as noted in Berke et al. (2010).

[4]   Individual studies of satisfaction for amputees can be found in McFarland et al. (2010) for unilateral upper-limb loss, Gailey et al. (2010) for unilateral lower-limb loss, and Dougherty et al. (2010) for multiple traumatic limb loss.

[5]   The study noted:

> A number of possible reasons exist for the higher overall satisfaction ratings in participants from the OIF/OEF conflict. At the outset is the structure of the initial care and rehabilitation process from the battlefield to rehabilitation care at DOD facilities. Also, expansion to multidisciplinary care may affect overall rehabilitation and prosthetic satisfaction. Our survey included OIF/OEF participants who were at least 1 year from limb loss. The factors identified by study participants included their involvement in prosthetic selection, training, and maintenance. A number of advancements to prosthetic materials and components are available to OIF/OEF servicemembers/veterans that were not initially available following the Vietnam era. These may not have been uniformly offered to Vietnam veterans. Additionally, it appears that providing multiple prostheses with different components and allowing each servicemember to meet his or her rehabilitation potential further stimulates involvement in former and new physical activities. The participants' ages and being greater than 1 year from amputation to survey may affect study finding. (Berke et al., 2010, p. 368)

of the "availability of new types of prosthetic devices and the higher expectations of OIF/OEF" amputees (Reiber et al., 2010, p. 291).[6] Nevertheless, the study noted that "remarkably higher percent of OIF/OEF participants with major limb loss returned to Active Duty given the opportunities afforded by the DOD and the rehabilitation paradigm shift" (Reiber et al., 2010, p. 287).

A headline in *U.S. News and World Report*, "New Prosthetics Keep Amputee Soldiers on Active Duty; Technology Advances—and Strong Willpower—Have Allowed Some Injured Soldiers to Return to Battle" (Koebler, 2012), attributed much of the success in the Army's program to the tenacity soldiers and advancements in prosthetics. In fact, the Army has led in the development and employment of new prosthetics ever since the Civil War.[7] Historically, wars have often been a catalyst for rapid innovation, and since September 11, 2001, that includes the rapid innovation of prosthetics.[8] Today, research sponsored by DOD's Defense Advanced Research Projects Agency (DARPA),[9] the VA, and the National Institutes of Health (NIH) and advances by private companies worldwide in the fields of microprocessors, robotics, and artificial intelligence make state-of-the-art prosthetics available to military amputees (Wilson, 2013). An example of how these advances have been incorporated into new prosthetics

---

[6] "Specifically, the annual rejection rate for those with unilateral upper-limb loss is 19.7-fold higher, for unilateral lower-limb loss is 15.0-fold higher, and for multiple limb loss is 19.9-fold higher. The availability of new types of prosthetic devices and the higher expectations of OIF/OEF servicemembers and veterans may explain the higher rejection rates" (Reiber et al., 2010, p. 291).

[7] In 1862, Congress appropriated $15,000 and authorized the Army to issue artificial limbs. The program began in 1864, with 669 artificial legs and 339 arms, and by the third year more than 6,000 had been issued. Many amputees' stumps could not be adequately fitted with artificial limbs, particularly if the amputation had been performed near the hip or shoulder. In others, pressure on the stump caused great pain. Figg and Farrell-Beck (1993, p. 464) note that "problems such as noise, weight, and appearance, as well as cost, availability, tendency to damage clothing, and pain in wearing might have been deterrents for [some] veterans."

[8] Kevin Carroll, vice president of Hanger, a prosthetics company that has been in existence since 1861, makes the point:

> Unfortunately, when you have war, you have casualties, but with that comes innovation. Artificial joints are getting better at approximating the knee, elbow, wrist, and ankle, and microprocessors embedded in prostheses are able to pick up and adjust for impacts from walking, running, jumping, and climbing. The person doesn't have to worry about the prosthetic device; they're worrying about the task in front of them. . . . If they want to go back to be with their troops, that's an option for many soldiers these days. (Koebler, 2012)

[9] In 2006, DARPA started the Revolutionizing Prosthetics program with the goal to expand prosthetic arm options for military amputees. The DEKA Research and Development Corporation was funded to quickly develop an arm control system to market and, together with Johns Hopkins Applied Physics Laboratory as the system integrator and lead, to produce a fully neutrally integrated upper-extremity prosthesis. The prosthesis incorporated sensors for touch, temperature, vibration, and proprioception; a power that will allow extended use; and mechanical components that provide strength and environmental tolerance to heat, cold, water, humidity, dust, and so on. With this new prosthetic, an upper-extremity amputee would be able to feel and manipulate objects just like a person with a native hand. In December 2016, Walter Reed delivered the first two advanced "Luke" arms, or Life Under Kinetic Evolution, named for Luke Skywalker a charter is *Star Wars*. See Sanchez (2017), Johns Hopkins Applied Physics Laboratory (undated), and DARPA (2016).

widely used by OEF/OIF military amputees is the microprocessor knee, or the C-Leg, shown in Figure B.1.[10]

The C-Leg knee is able to "sense the conditions acting on the knee joint and . . . quickly make internal adjustments. . . . Valves open or close electronically to increase or decrease fluid flow through the knee's internal ports . . . to vary resistance to knee flexion or extension" (Kapp and Miller, 2009, p. 560). Results of a clinical trial study with 17 amputees "show a statistically significant improvement in subjects' ability to descend stairs; time required to descend a slope; sound side-step length while descending compared to a mechanical knee (Hafner et al., 2007, p. 216). While traditionally the C-Leg was given only to amputees who have proven their ability to walk, the USAAPCP at Walter Reed was "the first facility in the world to utilized [sic] it as a *rehabilitative knee unit*" (Miller, 2004, p. 1) by adjusting the microprocessor program as the patient progresses through rehabilitation.

The costs of advanced prosthetics are substantial; the C-Leg microprocessor knee shown in Figure B.1 was estimated to cost $58,000 in 2004; others cost as much as $87,000.[11] In 2010, the VA projected future lifetime costs for OIF/OEF service members with unilateral upper-limb loss to be $823,239, with unilateral lower-limb loss to be $1,463,624, with bilateral upper-limb loss to be $2,158,244, and other types of multiple limb loss to be $2,901,355 (Blough et al., 2010).

In addition to advancements in prosthetics, gait training also advanced when the Computer-Assisted Rehab Environment (CAREN) was introduced to providers and patients at MATC, CFI, and C5. The CAREN treadmill gait-training system is made up of an instrumented treadmill on a six degree-of-freedom motion base platform and a large flat, curved panoramic, or dome screen upon which a variety of scenes are projected, as shown in Figure B.2. The system allows the operator to generate visual and physical perturbations that require users to make dynamic changes to their gait patterns as they walk through the scenes, which are synchronized with the movements of the platform and patient. A three-dimensional motion capture system collects data

---

[10] The availability of the C-Leg at Walter Reed was noted in January 2005:

> I[n] an effort to provide best care to all returning soldiers, all lower limb amputees from Knee disarticulation to hip disarticulation receive a "C-Leg" manufactured by Otto Bock Healthcare Inc. As well as a conventional hydraulic designed prosthesis, which can be configured as a running prosthesis and finally water-use prosthesis. (Miller, 2004)

The VA, however, was not as enthusiastic about the C-Leg as was the USAAPCP. It thought further "research is needed to ascertain which commercially available prosthetic devices are appropriate for particular clinical needs," and noted that "a comparison of conventional knee systems (Mauch SNS) to microprocessor-controlled knees (C-Leg) has not been performed," and argued that "in light of the activity levels of amputees returning from Iraq and the high maintenance and delicate components of the C-Leg, soldiers may benefit more from a traditional SNS knee" (Scoville, 2004e, pp. 3, 5).

[11] See Scoville (2004d). In 2007, it was reported that the average cost of prosthetic devices at Walter Reed was $115,000 per patient (Scoville, 2007b).

Figure B.1
Microprocessor Knee

Getting out of the chair
The modern above-knee prosthesis, called the C-Leg, is a microprocessor-controlled marvel of metal and plastic. Introduced in the United States in 1999, this prosthesis is a vast improvement over earlier artificial legs, enhancing comfort, security, and freedom and the ability to continue with an active lifestyle.

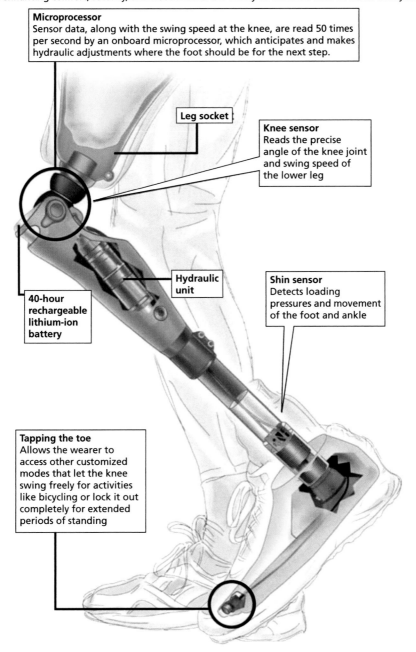

Microprocessor
Sensor data, along with the swing speed at the knee, are read 50 times per second by an onboard microprocessor, which anticipates and makes hydraulic adjustments where the foot should be for the next step.

Leg socket

Knee sensor
Reads the precise angle of the knee joint and swing speed of the lower leg

Hydraulic unit

Shin sensor
Detects loading pressures and movement of the foot and ankle

40-hour rechargeable lithium-ion battery

Tapping the toe
Allows the wearer to access other customized modes that let the knee swing freely for activities like bicycling or lock it out completely for extended periods of standing

SOURCE: SISSON Mobility Restoration Center, Inc.

on movement as the patient moves on the platform. The system costs in excess of $1 million.

The CAREN system

> allows a wounded warrior to be immersed in a realistic clinical environment, while therapist and physicians collect kinematic and kinetic data in order to plan future rehabilitation regimens. In everyday life, warfighters with lower extremity trauma may experience uneven terrain, cracks in pavements, slippery conditions, etc.—all potential scenarios that would may increase fall risk or injury. However, when using the CAREN system, specific physical perturbations may simulate these environmental conditions in a more safe and controlled setting. Depending on the warfighters' rehabilitation goals, simulations in the CAREN system may challenge reactive balance, reaction time, and muscle activation in order to improve gait and stability, obstacle avoidance or improved weight shifting. (Isaacson, Swanson, and Pasquina, 2013, p. 297)

Research has shown that CAREN can help train those with amputations to avoid falling by using their uninjured limb with little change in prosthetic ankle or knee kinematics on the affected side.[12] While traditional therapy methods will always have a place in the clinic, virtual reality–based gait-training programs can directly influence physiological and biomechanical performance. The CAREN system was also used to compare a number of different of prosthetic limbs: the conventional single axis hydraulic (SAH) knee, a two-microprocessor-controlled prosthetic (i.e., C-Leg), and the Genium X2 microprocessor knee during slope ambulation. The study showed that when descending a 10-degree slope the X2 users maintained a faster walking speed and took longer steps than those using either the SAH or C-Leg knee, and also did not require ambulatory aids.[13]

---

[12] See Werner, Linberg, and Wolf (2012).

[13] See Nottingham et al. (2012); Bell et al. (2016).

Figure B.2
Computer-Assisted Rehabilitation Environment

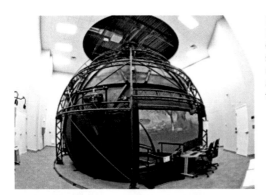

Motek Medical's Computer Assisted Rehabilitation Environment (CAREN) extended system is a virtual environment consisting of a 180-degree projection screen used to display a virtual scene, a 12-camera motion capture system, and a 6-degree-of-freedom actuated platform equipped with a dual-belt treadmill and two force plates.

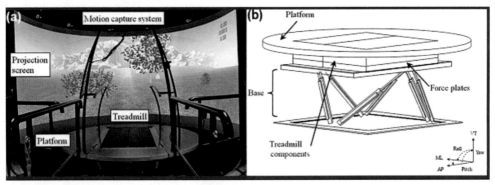

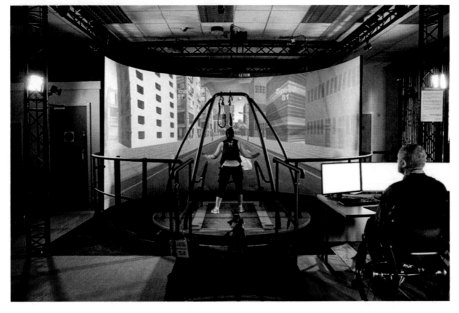

SOURCE: Top: Strive Center, homepage, undated; middle: Sinitski, Lemaire, and Baddour, 2015; bottom: Birchall Blackburn Law, undated.

Interview Guides

This appendix includes the guides that were used to interview providers and patients/family members. Each interview was conducted in person or over the phone, was semi-structured in nature, and lasted 45–60 minutes. The research team emailed potential interviewees to request their participation in a voluntary, confidential interview. At the beginning of each interview, a member of the RAND Arroyo Center research team verbally asked for the participant's consent to the interview and permission to record it (so it could later be transcribed and analyzed), and provided the individual with contact information for both RAND's Human Subject Protection Committee and the principal investigators.

Provider Interview Guide

Setting the Stage

1. Provider information—Please tell us a bit about yourself:
   - Background/Training
   - *Note to interviewer: Identify role of provider here to use throughout interview.*
   - Years of service (if military/former military)
   - Deployment experiences (if military/former military)
   - Experience with amputee rehabilitation care
   - Experience working at C5/CFI/WRNMMC (years working here, current military/civilian/contractor/prior experience in any of these categories)

Confirm primary provider role to be used for the interview

Understanding the role of the provider across the phases

Discuss handout about traumatic amputation phases. (RAND interviewer will explain that the interview is focused on understanding the provider's role in the five phases described in the handout, shown in Figure 1.2 of this report, which was adapted to reflect the Amputation Coalition's phases for traumatic amputations as opposed to delayed amputations).

Amputee care pathways *Note to interviewer: We are looking for skills/competencies as well as best practices that relate to amputee rehab care. For example, skill = knowing the right time to build and fit a prosthetic; best practice = having a case manager on staff to guide the patient through the phases.*

2. Can you tell me a little bit about what your role and activities are across these five phases from postoperative care to reintegration? *Note to interviewer: Okay if respondent wants to talk about the two phases not in our immediate focus (especially preoperative) as this may provide additional context for his/her role in other phases. Probe for details as time permits.*
    a. Probe for what other providers the respondent works with during each phase, and what that working relationship looks like in practice. Probe for any challenges with the described working relationship. *Note to interviewer: Okay to ask about skills as a whole after the respondent describes his/her role in each phase, as long as you probe for differences in how important different skills are perceived to be in each phase.*
    b. Probe for if/how the respondent works with the patient's family (e.g., Do you work with the patient only or with the family also? In what ways?).
    c. As the respondent describes his/her role in each phase, probe for what specific skills are perceived to be important/helpful to have in each of the phases. *Note to interviewer: As you are learning about skills, try to start developing a list of skills the provider says he/she needs.*

Drilling down into the specific skills that are important

3. When you think about an effective [nurse, physician, therapist, psychologist, etc.], what types of skills, behaviors, or personalities makes those people effective at Walter Reed? *Note to interviewer: Again, focus on skills/behaviors the participant discusses and add to the list you're creating.*
4. (*List the skills the provider said he/she needs and those needed to be effective.*) What skills are we missing?
5. You've described several different skills for us; can you tell us how do people generally learn these skills, or how do they get good at them? (*Probe for sources such as medical school, OJT [on-the-job training], mentorship, conferences, journals, other.*)
6. What are skills that cut across all rehabilitation providers hired at Walter Reed that they must have to be successful here?
7. How prepared were you when you started/what was challenging/what did you need?

Identifying skills at risk for atrophy and opportunities for maintenance

8. As the military amputee patient flow starts to slow, what knowledge/skills/abilities are you worried will atrophy?
9. How can you sustain those skills? Training? Other patient populations? *Note to interviewer: Probe for what's unique about the military population. Is working for military amputee different than civilian, or is it one limb vs. multiple limbs? What's really different that would be important to train up on? Does limb salvage provide practice for amputee rehab?*
    a. Probe for how differences in patient populations can contribute to or detract from skills maintenance—e.g., military vs. civilian amputee; single vs. multiple amputation; traumatic vs. conventional amputation; combat-related vs. deployment-related vs. neither.
10. To what extent are the skills that you use/think are important to amputee rehab care unique to the military population (versus skills that are generalizable across amputee populations). *Note to interviewer: Ask this if answer is not provided above.*

Patient/Family Member Interview Guide

Note to Interviewer: If the patient/family member seems uncomfortable during the interview, we need to ask whether we should stop the interview, and if that happens, we should also offer a resource the patient/family member can call to discuss his/her feelings.

1. *Note to interviewer: Do not go into etiology of injury directly; it might come up naturally in the flow of the discussion but we do not want to make the participant relive the experience.* To begin with, can you tell us a little bit about yourself; for example, how long have you served in the military (*probe for current status as still serving versus medically retired, if appropriate*) and where you have deployed? *Note to interviewer: If the interviewee is not currently serving, he/she can be offered a $50 Amazon gift card.*
    a. *Note to interviewer: If family member is present, or is the interviewee, probe relationship to amputee.*

As I briefly mentioned, we are here to better understand what kinds of skills, abilities, and knowledge providers should have in order to provide the best rehab services to amputees. This list [Figure 1.2 in this report] is how the Amputation Coalition describes the different phases of care involved in amputation rehabilitation, from pre-op (usually in the field at the point of injury) to maintenance or ongoing care beyond direct amputee rehab. (*Walk through with respondent.*)

2. Which phase of care would you say you are currently in?
3. We are interested in hearing an overview of the care you've received up to [the phase the participant identifies in # 2 above].
   a. Starting with the post-op phase, can you tell us where you received that care? Was it all at Walter Reed/CFI/C5 or VA or elsewhere?
      i. Which types of providers took care of you during the post-op phase? *Note to interviewer: Try to create a list of all providers who were relevant for each of these phases.*
      ii. What did they do specifically that was helpful for you? (*Go through list you created in 3a above.*)
      iii. What were the most important skills [name each specific provider] used when helping you in this phase?
      iv. Did these providers work with you one-on-one or did different providers work together (example, PT and OT [occupational therapist] collaborating) in treating you?
      v. [If they worked together], can you describe what their working together looked like? What did they do to work together? *Note to interviewer: Repeat this for the all phases the patient has experienced, up to and including reintegration if appropriate. Can also probe with the questions below:*
         • Can you describe for us the extent to which your care was delivered by teams vs. individual providers? (*Probe for number and types of providers, number and types of teams, effectiveness of coordination.*)
         • Did you feel that teams brought important skills to your rehabilitation beyond the skills that individual professionals brought?
   b. What services or procedures were helpful during the post-op phases (i.e., introduction to someone from the peer visitor program)?
4. Which parts of your rehab experience have been the most help for you to achieve or make progress toward your [or your loved one's] goals? Which providers were involved and in what ways? What was something really memorable about a provider that made your care or experience better? What was especially positive?
5. What characteristics do good providers have?
6. What are skills that ALL providers at Walter Reed must have when working with patients who are rehabilitating after an amputation?
7. If you received care from different types of providers, can you describe any challenges you encountered in going from one setting/provider to another (e.g., moving from PT to psychology)?
8. If you received care at different facilities, can you describe any challenges you encountered in going from one facility to another (e.g., moving from Landstuhl in Germany to Walter Reed/CFI/C5 or between DOD and VA)?
9. What parts of your rehabilitation could have been improved and in what ways? (*Probe for additional services needed.*)

10. [For family member specifically, if present] How would you describe the support that you received over the course of your patient's rehabilitation?
   a. Which providers did you interact with most closely?
   b. Which providers helped you the most as you helped your patient recover and rehabilitate?
   c. Did you have a sense as to what your needs are/were, and to what extent were they met?
   d. What additional services, or service improvements, would have improved your experience?

Codebook for Qualitative Analysis

Table D.1
Codebook for Qualitative Analysis

Code	Definition with Examples
Phase (code when the specific phase is explicitly mentioned or when the specific phase or implicitly described)	
Phase 1: Preoperative	Any mention of roles, care tasks or other activities occurring during the operative phase—i.e., immediately before or during or related to definitive surgery; essentially, anything that is after point of injury/theater but before the post-op phase
Phase 2: Postoperative	Any mention of roles, care tasks or other activities happening immediately after definitive surgery and focused on surgical recovery; most wound care occurs here
Phase 3: Preprosthetic	Any mention of roles, care tasks or other activities happening once surgical recovery is well under way or near complete, and preparation for a prosthetic has begun—e.g., shrinking, wrapping, limb strengthening, limb desensitization, fitting a test socket, making the prosthetic
Phase 4: Preparatory Prosthetic Training	Any mention of roles, care tasks, or other activities happening once patient begins to use prosthesis, including basic prosthetic skills, early weight bearing, and initial gait training
Phase 5: Definitive Prosthetic Training	Any mention of roles, care tasks, or other activities happening once patient is actively using prosthesis and able to intensify rehab goals with the prosthesis; focused on developing individualized treatment plans and getting to individual functional outcomes
Phase 6: Reintegration	Any mention of roles, care tasks, or other activities happening once the patient is regularly using a prosthesis and reintegrating into routine life—e.g., resumption of family and community roles, resumption of previous and adapted vocational and recreational activities
Phase 7: Maintenance/Ongoing Care	Any mention of roles, care tasks, or other activities taking place beyond amputee rehab care—e.g., follow-up visits, refittings, after being discharged from amputee rehab care

Table D.1—Continued

Code	Definition with Examples
Roles/Tasks (code when respondent is describing what he/she does in terms of amputee rehab care)	
Medical Care	Most direct patient care, including surgical care, wound care, pain management, comorbid management, limb desensitization; also includes PT/OT work such as help with basic activities of daily living (ADLs) (bathing, eating, dressing) and other physical rehab work including things like gait training
Behavioral Health Care	Behavioral health interventions, including psychological counseling, spiritual care
Reintegration Support	Training and support in terms of reintegration; helping patients with socialization, sports, navigating public spaces
Social Services/Case Management	Assistance with setting up housing, getting military pay, making referrals, connecting patients to resources
Patient/Family Education/Training or Support	Educating patient and/or family on amputee care activities (e.g., wound self-management, wrapping), setting and managing expectations with patients/families, communicating with families, providing support to family members
Clinical Team Coordination/ Communication	Role as it relates to communications, interactions, coordination with/between individual rehab team members, full rehab team, or other services/teams
Knowledge or Skills (code when respondent is describing specific skills or knowledge needed or used to provide amputee rehab care)	
KS	Knowledge or skills that are used or needed by amputee care professionals, described generally, as specific to amputee care, or as specific to a certain discipline or role
KS: Specific to Military	Knowledge or skills pertaining to being in the military; knowledge of military culture in the context of amputee care
KS: Gaps	Critical gaps in needed knowledge/skills—i.e., a knowledge or skill perceived as necessary but lacking
KS: Acquisition or Maintenance	How knowledge or skills are acquired or maintained
KS: Atrophy	Specific knowledge or skills at risk of atrophy in the context of a drawdown or decline in volume
Other	
Opportunities for Improvement	Wishes expressed by the respondent regarding what could make amputee care better

Table D.1—Continued

Code	Definition with Examples
Interdisciplinary Team-Based Care	Amputee care in the context of teams, including the importance of team-based care, critical members of the team, or barriers/facilitators to providing team-based care (e.g., inadequate staffing, team dynamics/interpersonal dynamics, patient volume). This may be double-coded with ROLES: Clinical team coordination/communication. Note that "team-based care" may or may not be talked about in the general context of amputee care, but rather than in terms of the respondent's roles or tasks.
Best Practices	Features, processes, or structures that facilitate optimal amputee rehab care and might be considered for translation to other centers/settings/units
Respondent Background	Description of respondent's training, military experience, background at the site, other places worked, etc.
Historical Context	Background/context to amputee care in the military, historical context of the site (not background about the provider, but background about the system or setting)
Amputation Type	Provider or patient discussing a specific type of amputation
Interesting	Do not use in combination with other codes. Use only for ideas/concepts that are potentially relevant to our study, but not captured by any other code

Results of the Technical Expert Survey

Within these tables, the behaviors are presented within each of the six competencies described above. We present the mean importance, mean frequency, and weighted criticality scores for each of the behaviors, with behaviors sorted according to weighted critical score (with highest scores appearing first). In addition, we highlight which behaviors reached consensus after the two rounds of surveys (labeled "high agreement" in the table), as well as those for which there was still a lack of agreement (labeled "low agreement").

Table E.1
Behavioral Health Technical Expert Survey on Competencies for Amputation Rehabilitation

	Mean Importance	Mean Frequency	Weighted Criticality Score
Competency: Teamwork			
High Agreement			
Use empathy, reflection, and interpersonal skills to effectively engage with other health professionals and members of the rehabilitation team.	4.8	4.6	14.2
Effectively call on other resources in the health care system to provide optimal health care.[c]	4.6	4.0	13.2
Effectively communicate and collaborate with multidisciplinary team members.	4.4	4.4	13.2
Support the medical and surgical staff.	4.0	3.6	11.6
Low Agreement			
Use interprofessional collaboration as appropriate to provide effective rehabilitation services.[c]	4.6	4.2	13.4
Communicate results of assessments and recommendations to providers on care team.[c]	4.2	3.8	12.2
Competency: Patient and Family Education			
Low Agreement			
Educate family members about the process of rehabilitation and what to expect throughout the trajectory of recovery.[c]	4.2	3.8	12.2
Orient family to the rehabilitation process.[b]	3.8	3.2	10.8
Provide developmentally appropriate education and/or educational materials for children of amputees to help them better understand amputation and the rehabilitation process.[b]	3.4	2.8	9.6
Competency: Military and Other Cultural Awareness			
High Agreement			

Table E.1—Continued

	Mean Importance	Mean Frequency	Weighted Criticality Score
Apply self-awareness and self-regulation to manage the influence of personal biases and values in working with diverse clients.	4.4	4.0	12.8
Apply knowledge related to military culture.[c]	4.2	4.4	12.8
Apply awareness of diversity and multicultural factors at the individual and cultural level as related to disability.[c]	4.2	4.2	12.6
Apply awareness of the interaction between one's own individual and cultural diversity characteristics as it influences professional functioning.[c]	4.2	4.2	12.6
Low Agreement			
Demonstrate competence in the evaluation and treatment of patients from diverse backgrounds, including patients of different ages, genders, and ethnic, racial, sociocultural, and economic backgrounds.[c]	4.0	4.2	12.2
Competency: Patient-Centered Care			
High Agreement			
Be responsive to patient needs in a way that supersedes self-interest.	4.8	4.6	14.2
Foster a therapeutic alliance with the patient.	4.8	4.6	14.2
Use empathy, reflection, and interpersonal skills to effectively engage with clients/patients and family members.	4.6	4.6	13.8
Demonstrate acceptance, compassion, integrity, respect, warmth, advice, praise, affirmation, and a sense of hope while working with patients.	4.6	4.4	13.6
Connect with the patient so that the patient sees the provider as a healthy adjunct to his or her recovery.	4.6	4.2	13.4
Understand the emotional impact of an injury, both in terms of the acute event and the ongoing emotional trauma that accompanies the change in body image and loss of function.	4.6	4.2	13.4
Demonstrate sensitivity to the welfare, rights, and dignity of others.	4.4	4.4	13.2

Table E.1—Continued

	Mean Importance	Mean Frequency	Weighted Criticality Score
Provide patient care that is compassionate, appropriate, and effective for the treatment of health problems and the promotion of health.	4.4	4.4	13.2
Strive to reduce unnecessary stressors for patients.[c]	4.4	4.4	13.2
Negotiate, mediate, advocate, and facilitate effective care transitions.[c]	4.6	3.8	13.0
Develop mutually agreed-on intervention goals and objectives based on the critical assessment of strengths, needs, and challenges with the patient.	4.2	4.4	12.8
Act as a patient advocate.	4.2	4.2	12.6
Provide support to patients, beyond the implementation of specific therapeutic techniques.[c]	4.2	4.2	12.6
Treat the whole patient, rather than providing symptom-focused treatment.	4.2	3.8	12.2
Manage patient expectations during the rehabilitation process.	4.0	4.2	12.2
Present self as a learner and engage clients and constituencies as experts of their own experiences.[c]	4.0	4.2	12.2
Select appropriate intervention strategies based on the assessment, research knowledge, and values and preferences of patients.	4.0	4.2	12.2
Collaborate with the patient to identify a treatment goal.	4.0	4.2	12.2
Work with patients to set realistic rehabilitation expectations.[b]	4.0	4.2	12.2
Assist patients with identifying recovery and rehabilitation goals to cultivate motivation for getting better.[b]	4.0	4.2	12.2
Implement therapeutic interventions as related to adjustment to disability for patients.	4.0	4.0	12.0
Demonstrate knowledge and provide support for patients struggling with body image, self-esteem, and/or self-image.[b]	4.0	4.0	12.0
Low Agreement			

Table E.1—Continued

	Mean Importance	Mean Frequency	Weighted Criticality Score
Implement therapeutic interventions as related to adjustment to disability for family members.[c]	4.2	3.8	12.2
Serve as a liaison between families and medical and support staff.[c]	4.2	3.6	12.0
Apply knowledge of human behavior and social environment, person-in-environment, and other multidisciplinary theoretical frameworks to engage with clients and constituencies.[c]	3.6	4.0	11.2
Competency: Evidence-Based Practice			
High Agreement			
Integrate awareness of common comorbidities, such as traumatic brain injury, when developing and implementing a treatment plan.[c]	4.4	4.4	13.2
Diagnose and treat patients in outpatient settings.[a]	4.2	4.2	12.6
Provide individual interventions.[a]	4.2	4.2	12.6
Conduct assessments focused on the domains of educational and vocational capacities, personality and emotional adjustment, sexual functioning, pain, substance use/abuse, and social and behavioral functioning.	4.3	4.0	12.5
Apply knowledge of health behavior change and provide health behavior counseling (e.g., smoking cessation, physical activity, diet).[b]	4.2	4.0	12.4
Diagnose mental health disorders using reliable and valid diagnostic techniques.[c]	4.0	4.2	12.2
Collect and organize data and apply critical thinking to interpret information from clients and constituencies.	4.0	4.2	12.2
Demonstrate knowledge of adaptation to trauma, including stages of adaptation and how this influences care.[b]	4.0	4.2	12.2
Diagnose and treat patients in inpatient settings.[a]	3.6	4.0	11.2
Low Agreement			

Table E.1—Continued

	Mean Importance	Mean Frequency	Weighted Criticality Score
Participate in professional activities and continuing education relevant to rehabilitation and mental health.[c]	4.3	3.5	12.0
Utilize scientific and evidence-based theory to inform one's practice and professional functioning.[c]	4.0	3.8	11.8
Conduct assessments focused on the domains of adjustment to disability and extent and nature of disability and preserved abilities.[c]	4.0	3.8	11.8
Assess patient attitudes toward the amputation, including whether he or she was prepared for the need for the amputation.[b]	4.0	3.8	11.8
Evaluate patients prior to having an amputation to prepare the patient, identify potential psychosocial issues, and maximize outcomes.[c] (high importance low frequency)[b]	4.0	3.6	11.6
Utilize behavioral management strategies.[c]	3.8	4.0	11.6
Demonstrate awareness of phantom limb pain and behavioral treatments for phantom limb pain (e.g., hypnosis, mirror therapy).[c]	3.8	4.0	11.6
Identify and refer patients to peer support programs.[b]	3.8	3.8	11.4
Demonstrate basic knowledge of medical interventions and recovery from amputation (e.g., basic surgical knowledge, knowledge of wound healing and infections).[b]	3.8	3.8	11.4
Provide medication management, including identification of appropriate medication options and consideration of the patient's underlying medical condition, current medications, and allergies.[c]	3.6	4.0	11.2
Provide sexual counseling.[c]	3.8	3.3	10.8
Apply knowledge of evidence-based coping strategies.[c]	3.6	3.6	10.8
Conduct assessments focused on the domains of cognitive functioning and decisional capacity.[c]	3.6	3.4	10.6
Critically evaluate scientific and evidence-based theory and research.[c]	3.4	3.6	10.4
Provide group interventions.[a]	3.4	3.2	10.0

Table E.1—Continued

	Mean Importance	Mean Frequency	Weighted Criticality Score
Conduct routine screening evaluations to identify patients with behavioral health needs.[c]	3.0	3.8	9.8
Competency: Ethical and Professional Practice			
High Agreement			
Maintain appropriate boundaries and manage personal values in practice settings.	4.2	4.6	13.0
Demonstrate awareness of principles and practice standards, current statutory and state regulatory provisions, and issues related to patient confidentiality and privacy.	4.2	4.4	12.8
Demonstrate awareness of ethical principles and commitment to carrying out professional activities in a manner consistent with ethical guidelines.	4.2	4.4	12.8
Maintain professionalism in practice situations through behavior, appearance, and oral, written, and electronic communication.	3.8	4.4	12.0
Low Agreement			
Investigate and evaluate one's care of patients and continuously improve patient care based on constant self-evaluation.[c]	4.2	3.6	12.0
Maintain awareness of the effect that the work has on one's own mental health and well-being, and implement strategies to mitigate burnout (e.g., self-care).[c]	4.0	3.6	11.6
Demonstrate awareness of current issues facing the profession and implications to functioning as a behavioral health provider in a rehabilitation setting.[c]	3.8	3.8	11.4
Demonstrate awareness of the larger context and system of health care.[c]	3.8	3.8	11.4
Use supervision and consultation to guide professional adjustment and behavior.[c]	3.6	3.6	10.8
Demonstrate awareness and knowledge of laws related to Americans with Disabilities Act (ADA).[c]	3.4	3.2	10.0
Use technology ethically and appropriately to facilitate practice outcomes.[c]	3.2	3.4	9.8

Table E.1—Continued

NOTES:

[a] Reflects items that were part of a single item in round one but split into separate items in round two based on provider feedback.

[b] Indicates items that were proposed in the first survey and therefore were rated only once (in the second survey).

[c] Reflects items that had <70 percent agreement in the first survey.

IMPORTANCE scale ranges from 1 (not important) to 5 (critically important); frequency scale ranges from 1 (never) to 5 (all the time).

RESPONSES listed in table reflect the results of the second survey. If the item reached the agreement threshold after the second survey, it was no longer classified as low agreement.

Table E.2
Biomedical Engineering Technical Expert Survey on Competencies for Amputation Rehabilitation

	Mean Importance	Mean Frequency	Weight Criticality Score
Competency: Teamwork			
High Agreement			
Demonstrate the ability to communicate with different audiences (e.g., clinicians, researchers).	4.6	4.6	13.8
Collaborate with other providers on research protocols and studies to combine research lab resources and clinical needs.	3.8	4.2	11.8
Low Agreement			
Collaborate with other providers using an interdisciplinary approach to coordinate patient care.[c]	3.8	3.8	11.3
Educate clinicians on the role of engineers in amputee care, including what engineers do, why they are doing it, and what it means for clinical care.[b]	3.3	3.8	10.8
Perform evaluation and provide data analysis and reports for providers (e.g., prosthetists/orthotists) to inform care.[c]	3.8	3.0	10.5
Understand the broad scope of disciplines that support engineering theory and practice.[c]	2.8	3.3	8.8
Competency: Patient and Family Education			
High Agreement			
Translate research and engineering concepts in a way that patients and clinicians can understand.[b]	4.5	4.0	13.0
Clearly explain the complexity of technology or systems (e.g., CAREN), including the application and purpose.	3.8	4.2	11.8
Low Agreement			
Educate patients and family members on the role of engineers in amputee care, including what engineers do, why they are doing it, and what it means for their rehabilitation.[b]	3.5	3.0	10.0

Table E.2—Continued

	Mean Importance	Mean Frequency	Weight Criticality Score
Competency: Military and Other Cultural Awareness			
Low Agreement			
Demonstrate understanding of the way that military culture and military health system shape research.[c]	3.3	3.0	9.5
Demonstrate understanding of the way that military culture and the military health system shape clinical care.[c]	3.3	2.5	9.0
Demonstrate understanding of military culture and its influence on patient goals and milestones.[c]	3.0	2.3	8.3
Competency: Patient-Centered Care			
High Agreement			
Provide individualized care to patients.[c]	4.8	2.8	12.3
Competency: Evidence-Based Practice			
High Agreement			
Demonstrate knowledge of gait analysis.	4.6	4.4	13.6
Use a broad range of engineering tools, applications, and software.	4.4	4.8	13.6
Demonstrate general knowledge of computers and programming.	4.2	4.2	12.6
Combine knowledge of biological systems at the cellular and organ system level with quantitative analysis and core aspects of engineering.	3.2	2.8	9.2
Apply knowledge of engineering materials and their properties and behaviors.[c]	3.3	2.0	8.5
Understand the use and function of control systems.[c]	2.3	2.5	7.0
Demonstrate knowledge of power and energy systems fundamentals and their integration within the modern electrical grid and community.	1.4	1.6	4.4

Table E.2—Continued

	Mean Importance	Mean Frequency	Weight Criticality Score
Low Agreement			
Develop systems that are reliable and effective at mitigating risk and reducing failure.[c]	4.3	3.5	12.0
Gather requirements, develop models, and create prototypes in a timely and effective manner to increase a project's safety and success.[c]	3.8	3.0	10.5
Demonstrate familiarity with sensing and robotic technology.[b]	3.0	3.0	9.0
Solve thermodynamic engineering problems using mathematical formulations.[c]	2.0	1.8	5.8
Competency: Ethical and Professional Behavior			
High Agreement			
Behave in accordance with professional standards and ethics.	5.0	5.0	15.0
Demonstrate skills in research, such as data collection, protocol development, Institutional Review Board (IRB) applications, grant writing and applications, and publishing research results.	4.6	5.0	14.2

NOTES:
[b] Indicates items that were proposed in the first survey and therefore were rated only once (in the second survey).
[c] Reflects items that had <70 percent agreement in the first survey.

IMPORTANCE scale ranges from 1 (not important) to 5 (critically important); frequency scale ranges from 1 (never) to 5 (all the time). Responses listed in table reflect the results of the second survey. If the item reached the agreement threshold after the second survey, it is no longer classified as low agreement.

Table E.3
Case Management Technical Expert Survey on Competencies for Amputation Rehabilitation

	Mean Importance	Mean Frequency	Weighted Criticality Score
Competency: Teamwork			
High Agreement			
Facilitate coordination, communication, and collaboration with the patient and other stakeholders in order to achieve goals and maximize positive patient outcomes.	5.0	5.0	15.0
Communicate with all members of the multidisciplinary team.	5.0	5.0	15.0
Share information between providers and patient, especially regarding coverage and referrals.	5.0	5.0	15.0
Competency: Patient and Family Education			
High Agreement			
Provide education to family members.	4.8	5.0	14.5
Support family members.	4.8	4.8	14.3
Educate patients regarding their rehabilitative care.	4.8	4.8	14.3
Competency: Military and Other Cultural Awareness			
High Agreement			
Complete a health and psychosocial assessment, taking into account the cultural and linguistic needs of each patient.	4.8	5.0	14.5
Understand the disability system and how level of disability is connected to coverage of services (to maximize what the patient receives).	4.5	4.8	13.8
Demonstrate knowledge of VA, TRICARE/Medicare insurance, coverage levels, retirement disability, and other military-specific benefits.	4.5	4.5	13.5
Competency: Patient-Centered Care			

Table E.3—Continued

	Mean Importance	Mean Frequency	Weighted Criticality Score
High Agreement			
Identify immediate, short-term, long-term, and ongoing needs, as well as develop appropriate and necessary case management strategies and goals to address those needs.	5.0	5.0	15.0
Understand the clinical context in order to identify needed services.	5.0	5.0	15.0
Encourage and motivate the patient.	5.0	5.0	15.0
Advocate for patient's care.	5.0	4.8	14.8
Identify and remove gaps in the patient's care.	4.8	5.0	14.5
Demonstrate compassion and empathy for what the patient and his or her family are going through.	4.8	5.0	14.5
Identify and select patients who can most benefit from case management services available in a particular practice setting.	4.8	4.8	14.3
Coordinate community resources and services to support patient and family needs.[b]	4.8	4.8	14.3
Set patient expectations early and regularly throughout the rehab process.	4.7	4.7	14.0
Appropriately terminate case management services based upon the patient and other stakeholders in order to achieve goals and maximize positive client outcomes.	4.5	4.8	13.8
Identify issues occurring with the patient early and connect the patient with the right service.	4.5	4.5	13.5
Competency: Evidence-Based Practice			
High Agreement			
Maintain clinical skills within the discipline.	5.0	5.0	15.0
Collect background information about financial resources, education level, work history, living situation, and social support to help with treatment and discharge planning.	5.0	5.0	15.0

Table E.3—Continued

	Mean Importance	Mean Frequency	Weighted Criticality Score
Ensure that follow-up plans are implemented.	4.8	5.0	14.5
Identify problems or opportunities that would benefit from case management intervention.	4.8	4.8	14.3
Apply knowledge of mental health issues associated with limb loss (e.g., phantom limb pain, PTSD, altered body image).[b]	4.8	4.8	14.3
Demonstrate skills in addressing vocational transition, retraining, return-to-work, and/or return-to-active duty for patients following amputation.[b]	4.8	4.8	14.3
Demonstrate knowledge of different referral/authorization processes.	4.8	4.8	14.3
Maximize the patient's health, wellness, safety, adaptation, and self-care through quality case management, patient satisfaction, and cost-efficiency.	4.5	4.8	13.8
Employ ongoing assessment and documentation to measure the patient's response to the plan of care.	4.5	4.5	13.5
Coordinate equipment purchases.	4.3	4.3	12.8
Apply knowledge of home and vehicle modifications for wheelchair access.[b]	4.3	4.0	12.5
Apply knowledge of fitness and sports programs for patients post-rehabilitation.[b]	4.0	3.8	11.8
Apply knowledge of current prosthetic options and research in the areas of prosthetic fittings and technology.[b]	3.8	4.0	11.5
Low Agreement			
Apply knowledge of additional therapy modalities (e.g., art therapy, music therapy, animal-assisted therapy).[b]	4.0	4.3	12.3
Coordinate travel and housing as needed to off-site rehabilitation facilities that offer more comprehensive rehabilitation care.[b]	3.3	3.0	9.5
Competency: Ethical and Professional Behavior			

Table E.3—Continued

	Mean Importance	Mean Frequency	Weighted Criticality Score
High Agreement			
Maintain current, active, and unrestricted licensure or certification in health or human services discipline in order to conduct an assessment independently as permitted within the scope of practice of the discipline.	5.0	5.0	15.0
Adhere to applicable local, state, and federal laws and employer policies governing the patient, patient privacy, and confidentiality rights.	5.0	5.0	15.0
Obtain a baccalaureate or graduate degree from an accredited institution in social work or another health or human services field that promotes the physical, psychosocial, and/or vocational well-being of the persons being served.	4.8	4.5	14.0
Demonstrate a sense of humor and maturity when providing care.[b]	4.5	4.5	13.5

NOTES:
[b] Indicates items that were proposed in the first survey and therefore were rated only once (in the second survey).
[c] Reflects items that had <70 percent agreement in the first survey.

IMPORTANCE scale ranges from 1 (not important) to 5 (critically important); frequency scale ranges from 1 (never) to 5 (all the time). Responses listed in table reflect the results of the second survey. If the item reached the agreement threshold after the second survey, it is no longer classified as low agreement.

Table E.4
Diet and Nutrition Technical Expert Survey on Competencies for Amputation Rehabilitation

	Mean Importance	Mean Frequency	Weighted Criticality Score
Competency: Teamwork			
High Agreement			
Educate other providers on the role and importance of nutrition.	4.3	3.5	12.0
Low Agreement			
Implement community-based and population-based programs and/or interventions in collaboration with stakeholders.[c]	4.0	3.0	11.0
Collaborate with other providers to develop a targeted comprehensive rehabilitation plan.[c]	3.7	2.7	10.0
Collaborate with others to achieve common goals and to optimize delivery of services.[c]	3.3	2.7	9.3
Utilize appropriate communication methods and skills to meet the needs of providers.[c]	3.3	2.7	9.3
Employ strategies to facilitate team-building skills.[c]	2.7	1.7	7.0
Competency: Patient and Family Education			
High Agreement			
Utilize appropriate communication methods and skills to meet the needs of patients and family members.	4.8	3.8	13.3
Low Agreement			
Teach, guide, and instruct a variety of individuals, groups, or populations.[c]	4.7	3.3	12.7
Design, select, and implement education strategies to meet the learning needs of the individual, group, community, and population.[c]	3.7	3.0	10.3
Evaluate learning, including teaching style and delivery, using appropriately designed instruments.[c]	3.7	2.0	9.3
Establish, develop, and implement program outlines and learning plans to meet the needs of patients.[c]	3.3	2.3	9.0

Table E.4—Continued

	Mean Importance	Mean Frequency	Weighted Criticality Score
Competency: Military and Other Cultural Awareness			
Low Agreement			
Understand military-specific attitudes toward overall rehabilitation (e.g., athletic/competitive).[c]	4.7	3.7	13.0
Understand the science of nutrition in the context of sports medicine.[c]	4.3	3.7	12.3
Recognize and respect the physical, social, cultural, institutional, and economic environments of the individual, group, community, and population in practice.[c]	4.0	3.3	11.3
Competency: Patient-Centered Care			
High Agreement			
Increase patient self-efficacy.	5.0	4.0	14.0
Help patients set and meet personalized goals.	5.0	4.0	14.0
Demonstrate empathy.	4.8	4.0	13.5
Apply patient-centered principles in practice.	4.8	4.0	13.5
Adapt to the range of patient needs encountered in amputee care (e.g., be able to think outside the box when developing nutrition plan).	4.8	3.8	13.3
Motivate patients to adhere to nutrition regimens.	4.5	3.5	12.5
Advocate for proper nutrition with providers and patients.	4.3	3.8	12.3
Implement the Nutrition Care Process to ensure individual health goals are established, monitored, and achieved while adhering to the standards of practice for nutrition care.	4.3	3.8	12.3
Advocate for the patient and facilitate acquisition of services and resources.	3.8	3.3	10.8
Low Agreement			

Table E.4—Continued

	Mean Importance	Mean Frequency	Weighted Criticality Score
Engage patient or substitute decisionmaker in the informed consent process prior to and during the provision of services.[c]	4.3	3.7	12.3
Competency: Evidence-Based Practice			
High Agreement			
Stay current with the latest knowledge in nutrition (in general, and specific to amputee care).	4.8	3.8	13.3
Demonstrate a commitment to maintaining and enhancing knowledge.	4.5	4.0	13.0
Assess caloric and nutritional needs.	4.5	3.5	12.5
Apply knowledge of the interrelationship and impact of pharmacotherapy, dietary supplements, functional foods, and nutrients on health and disease in accordance with the scope of practice and standards of professional performance for dietitians/nutritionists.	4.5	3.5	12.5
Demonstrate sound professional judgment and strategic thinking in practice.	4.3	3.8	12.3
Recognize and apply education and learning theories and principles in practice.	4.3	3.5	12.0
Demonstrate skills in researching, independent critical examination, and evaluating literature to influence practice.	4.3	3.3	11.8
Interpret and apply current food and nutrition science and principles in dietetics practice.	4.0	3.3	11.3
Use effective counseling and coaching skills and strategies in practice.	4.0	3.3	11.3
Low Agreement			
Understand the role that nutritional support plays in achieving successful wound closure and wound healing.[c]	5.0	3.7	13.7
Perform nutrition screening to evaluate individual health, malnutrition, and disease while adhering to standards of practice in nutrition care.[c]	5.0	3.7	13.7

Table E.4—Continued

	Mean Importance	Mean Frequency	Weighted Criticality Score
Capture body measurements (e.g., waist-to-thigh ratio, limb length).[c]	5.0	3.3	13.3
Reflect, integrate, and evaluate using critical thinking when faced with problems, issues, and challenges.[c]	4.0	3.3	11.3
Evaluate nutrition programs to measure program effectiveness and outcomes and recommend modifications to support changes and/or sustainability of program.[c]	4.0	3.0	11.0
Assess the need to develop and implement community or population health programs and/or interventions.[c]	3.7	2.7	10.0
Develop a community and population health program or intervention to meet the needs of the community and/or population.[c]	3.7	2.7	10.0
Demonstrate and apply knowledge of culinary practices to effect behavioral change, taking into consideration client needs and demands.[c]	3.0	2.7	8.7
Use evidence-based literature and research to support the marketing, advertising, and sales of products and services.[c]	3.0	1.7	7.7
Analyze, design, and monitor food service systems to optimize operations.[c]	2.3	1.7	6.3
Competency: Ethical and Professional Behavior			
High Agreement			
Adhere to confidentiality and privacy legislation, standards, and policies.	5.0	4.0	14.0
Identify, analyze, and manage risk and adverse events to ensure safety to self, staff, client, and public.	4.8	4.0	13.5
Identify with and adhere to the code of ethics for the profession.	4.5	4.0	13.0
Integrate policies for and adhere to infection prevention and control measures.	4.5	4.0	13.0
Work within personal and professional limitations and abilities.	4.3	4.0	12.5
Adhere to and model professional obligations defined in legislation, standards, and organization policies.	3.5	3.8	10.8

Table E.4—Continued

	Mean Importance	Mean Frequency	Weighted Criticality Score
Develop, direct, manage, and evaluate the use of standardized recipes for food production in delivery systems.	2.0	1.8	5.8
Apply principles of project management to achieve goals and objectives.	2.0	1.8	5.8
Incorporate key sales principles while maintaining integrity of self, the organization, and the nutrition and dietetics profession.	2.0	1.5	5.5
Apply principles of financial management to support and achieve budgetary goals.	2.0	1.5	5.5
Coordinate human resource activities while adhering to labor agreements, organization policies, and applicable legislation.	1.5	1.5	4.5
Develop, manage, and demonstrate accountability for operational budgets in food service systems.	1.0	1.3	3.3
Low Agreement			
Document and maintain records according to standards of practice, legislation, regulations, and organization policies.[c]	4.7	3.3	12.7
Demonstrate resilience with challenging patients.[c]	4.3	3.0	11.7
Demonstrate and apply leadership skills.[c]	4.0	3.0	11.0
Utilize technology according to organization needs and workplace policies and procedures.[c]	4.0	3.0	11.0
Demonstrate ethical and professional behavior when using technology.[c]	3.7	3.3	10.7
Develop advertising messages and materials in a professional and ethical manner.[c]	3.7	3.0	10.3
Advocate for health and disease prevention in the community and population.[c]	3.7	3.0	10.3
Employ principles of productivity to optimize safe, ethical, and efficient resource utilization.[c]	3.7	2.7	10.0
Responsibly apply the principles of financial stewardship and/or management.[c]	3.7	2.7	10.0

Table E.4—Continued

	Mean Importance	Mean Frequency	Weighted Criticality Score
Demonstrate the ability to store and retrieve data using the International Dietetics and Nutrition Terminology (IDNT) and other standardized languages.[c]	3.3	3.0	9.7
Apply principles, standards, regulations, and organization policies to reduce the risk of foodborne and waterborne illness outbreaks.[c]	3.3	3.0	9.7
Lead or participate in the development of products and/or services related to food, nutrition, equipment, and systems.[c]	2.7	2.3	7.7
Participate in and/or lead research initiatives following ethical and professional research methodology.[c]	2.7	2.3	7.7
Lead, manage, and/or participate in quality improvement and customer satisfaction activities to improve delivery of services.[c]	3.0	1.7	7.7
Advocate and challenge others to take action to advance the profession.[c]	2.0	2.3	6.3

NOTES:
[b] Indicates items that were proposed in the first survey and therefore were rated only once (in the second survey).
[c] Reflects items that had <70 percent agreement in the first survey.

IMPORTANCE scale ranges from 1 (not important) to 5 (critically important); frequency scale ranges from 1 (never) to 5 (all the time). Responses listed in table reflect the results of the second survey. If the item reached the agreement threshold after the second survey, it is no longer classified as low agreement.

Table E.5
Occupational Therapy Technical Expert Survey on Competencies for Amputation Rehabilitation

	Mean Importance	Mean Frequency	Weighted Criticality Score
Competency: Teamwork			
High Agreement			
Collaborate with multidisciplinary team members to establish patient goals.	5.0	4.8	14.8
Coordinate the development and implementation of the occupational therapy intervention with the intervention provided by other professionals, when appropriate.	4.8	4.5	14.0
Collaborate with providers from other specialties to develop and implement a treatment plan.	4.5	4.5	13.5
Collaborate with prosthetists to identify electrode sites for myoelectric prostheses.	4.5	4.3	13.3
Recommend additional consultations or refer clients to appropriate resources when the needs of the client can best be served by the expertise of other professionals or services.	4.5	4.3	13.3
Educate current and potential referral sources about the scope of occupational therapy services and the process of initiating occupational therapy services.	4.3	4.5	13.0
Coordinate reintegration programs with other providers to facilitate transition to community life.	4.5	4.0	13.0
Competency: Patient and Family Education			
High Agreement			
Educate patients and help them to set realistic expectations about prostheses.	5.0	4.8	14.8
Teach patients and family members to don and doff compression garments, conduct limb massage and desensitization, and other postoperative tasks.	4.8	4.8	14.3
Teach patients how to use adaptive aids and compensatory techniques.	4.8	4.8	14.3
Educate family members so that they can assist the patient in implementing skills at home.	4.3	3.8	12.3
Competency: Military and Other Cultural Awareness			

Table E.5—Continued

	Mean Importance	Mean Frequency	Weighted Criticality Score
High Agreement			
Respect the patient's sociocultural background.	4.0	4.3	12.3
Understand the unique needs and preferences of a military patient population with regard to rehabilitation.	4.0	4.0	12.0
Competency: Patient-Centered Care			
High Agreement			
Collaborate with patients to set treatment goals.	5.0	5.0	15.0
Provide patient-centered and family-centered occupational therapy services.	4.8	5.0	14.5
Evaluate the patient's ability to participate in daily life by considering his or her history, goals, capacities, and needs, the activities and occupations the patient wants and needs to perform, and the environments and context in which these activities and occupations occur.	4.8	5.0	14.5
Garner patient buy-in for treatment and therapy.	4.8	5.0	14.5
Build rapport and establish a therapeutic relationship with patients.	4.8	5.0	14.5
Apply problem-solving skills and innovation to provide effective treatment.	5.0	4.5	14.5
Engage in expectation management with patients and family members.	4.8	4.8	14.3
Help patients gain independence in self-care and a sense of control over environment.	4.8	4.5	14.0
Collaborate with the patient to develop and implement the intervention plan, on the basis of the patient's needs and priorities, safety issues, and relative benefits and risks of the interventions.	4.5	4.8	13.8
Prepare and implement a transition or discontinuation plan based on the patient's needs, goals, performance, and appropriate follow-up resources.	4.5	4.5	13.5

Table E.5—Continued

	Mean Importance	Mean Frequency	Weighted Criticality Score
Modify the intervention plan throughout the intervention process and document changes in the patient's needs, goals, and performance.	4.3	4.8	13.3
Understand patient motivations, interests, and level of commitment.	4.3	4.6	13.3
Select, measure, document, and interpret expected or achieved outcomes that are related to the patient's ability to engage in occupations.	4.5	4.3	13.3
Transition the patient to other types or intensity of service or discontinue services when the patient has achieved identified goals, reached maximum benefit, or does not desire to continue services.	4.3	4.5	13.0
Facilitate the transition or discharge process in collaboration with the patient, family members, significant others, other professionals (e.g., medical, educational, or social services), and community resources when appropriate.	4.3	4.3	12.8
Provide psychological support to patients and family members.	4.3	4.3	12.8
Be adaptable in the approach to treatment.	4.3	4.0	12.6
Approach rehabilitation in a creative manner to best meet the needs of patients.	4.0	4.5	12.5
Competency: Evidence-Based Practice			
High Agreement			
Develop and implement the occupational therapy intervention based on the evaluation, patient goals, best available evidence, and professional and clinical reasoning.	4.5	5.0	14.0
Conduct comprehensive evaluations of patients at the beginning of rehabilitation, including functional abilities, range of motion, wound description, and pain.	4.5	4.8	13.8
Apply knowledge of specific rehabilitation techniques, such as postural exercises and strengthening, muscle strengthening and endurance.	4.5	4.3	13.3
Implement clinical interventions, including range of motion training, ADL training, and wound care.	4.3	4.5	13.0

Table E.5—Continued

	Mean Importance	Mean Frequency	Weighted Criticality Score
Implement nonpharmacological pain management strategies (e.g., transcutaneous baths, functional tasks to encourage normal motor pattern, desensitization).	4.3	4.0	12.5
Apply knowledge of polytrauma and common comorbidities and the effect on treatment.	4.3	4.0	12.5
Use current assessments and assessment procedures.	4.0	4.3	12.3
Follow defined protocols of standardized assessments during the screening, evaluation, and reevaluation process.[c]	4.0	4.0	12.0
Apply knowledge of anatomy and physiology.	4.0	4.0	12.0
Apply evidence-based research ethically and appropriately to provide occupational therapy services consistent with best practice approaches.	3.8	4.3	11.8
Apply knowledge of new technologies and advancements in care.	3.8	4.3	11.8
Conduct prehension evaluations.	3.3	3.0	9.5
Competency: Ethical and Professional Behavior			
High Agreement			
Maintain current licensure, registration, or certification as required by law or regulation.	5.0	5.0	15.0
Abide by the Occupational Therapy Code of Ethics.	5.0	5.0	15.0
Be accountable for the safety and effectiveness of the occupational therapy service delivery process.	5.0	5.0	15.0
Be self-motivated and self-directed.	4.8	5.0	14.5
Deliver occupational therapy services in accordance with American Occupational Therapy Association (AOTA) standards, policies, and guidelines and state, federal, and other regulatory and payer requirements relevant to practice and service delivery.	4.8	4.8	14.3
Demonstrate responsibility for all aspects of occupational therapy service delivery.	4.5	5.0	14.0

Table E.5—Continued

	Mean Importance	Mean Frequency	Weighted Criticality Score
Demonstrate attention to detail.	4.5	4.8	13.8
Demonstrate responsibility for all aspects of the screening, evaluation, and reevaluation process.	4.3	4.8	13.3
Deliver services that reflect the philosophical base of occupational therapy and are consistent with the established principles and concepts of theory and practice.	4.3	4.5	13.0
Establish, maintain, and update professional performance, knowledge, and skills.	4.0	4.8	12.8
Document services within the time frames, formats, and standards established by practice settings, federal and state law, other regulatory and payer requirements, external accreditation programs, and AOTA documents.	4.0	4.8	12.8
Use knowledge of outside and community-based resources available to patients and families.	4.5	3.8	12.8
Communicate screening, evaluation, and reevaluation results within the boundaries of client confidentiality and privacy regulations to the appropriate person, group, organization, or population.	4.3	4.0	12.5
Low Agreement			
Maintain current knowledge of legislative, political, social, cultural, societal, and reimbursement issues that affect patients and the practice of occupational therapy.[c]	3.6	3.6	11.0

NOTES:
[b] Indicates items that were proposed in the first survey and therefore were rated only once (in the second survey).
[c] Reflects items that had <70 percent agreement in the first survey.

IMPORTANCE scale ranges from 1 (not important) to 5 (critically important); frequency scale ranges from 1 (never) to 5 (all the time). Responses listed in table reflect the results of the second survey. If the item reached the agreement threshold after the second survey, it is no longer classified as low agreement.

Table E.6
Orthopaedic Surgery Technical Expert Survey on Competencies for Amputation Rehabilitation

	Mean Importance	Mean Frequency	Weighted Criticality Score
Competency: Teamwork			
High Agreement			
Use interpersonal and communication skills that result in the effective exchange of information and collaboration with health professionals.	4.5	5.0	14.0
Effectively call on other resources in the system to provide optimal health care.	4.0	4.3	12.3
Low Agreement			
Work together with providers from other disciplines.[c]	4.0	4.7	12.7
Collaborate with the rehabilitation team to develop care plans.[c]	3.7	4.3	11.7
Collaborate with other providers prior to amputation surgery, including other surgeons and allied professions (e.g., prosthetist).[c]	3.0	3.3	9.3
Competency: Patient and Family Education			
No items.			
Competency: Military and Other Cultural Awareness			
Low Agreement			
Demonstrate sensitivity and responsiveness to a diverse patient population, including but not limited to diversity in gender, age, culture, race, religion, disabilities, and sexual orientation.[c]	3.7	4.7	12.0
Have ability to manage the emotional aspects associated with the treatment of combat trauma.[c]	4.0	4.3	12.3
Competency: Patient-Centered Care			
High Agreement			

Table E.6—Continued

	Mean Importance	Mean Frequency	Weighted Criticality Score
Interpersonal and communication skills that result in the effective exchange of information and collaboration with patients and their families.	4.8	4.8	14.3
Provide patient care that is compassionate, appropriate, and effective for the treatment of health problems and the promotion of health.	4.3	5.0	13.5
Communicate rehabilitation and functional expectations with patients when developing a surgical care plan.	4.5	4.5	13.5
Provide counseling to patients and families to establish realistic expectations regarding medical aspects of recovery (e.g., risk of infection).	4.5	4.5	13.5
Consider the potential functional rehabilitation of the entire patient when addressing limb salvage versus amputation or residual limb length decisions.	4.3	4.8	13.3
Work cooperatively with the patient and family to develop care plans.	4.3	4.8	13.3
Competency: Evidence-Based Practice			
High Agreement			
Apply knowledge of surgical techniques, including preservation of tissue, nerve management, and open wound management.	5.0	5.0	15.0
Apply understanding of the different surgical considerations for upper versus lower extremity amputations.	4.8	4.8	14.3
Apply understanding of medical and surgical management of infection following amputation.[c]	4.7	5.0	14.3
Apply understanding of soft tissue injuries that result from combat trauma.[c]	4.7	5.0	14.3
Apply understanding of surgical management of neuromas.	4.5	5.0	14.0
Understand prosthetic options for different amputation levels.[b]	4.3	5.0	13.7
Apply understanding of principles related to definitive closure and debridement.	4.5	4.5	13.5

Table E.6—Continued

	Mean Importance	Mean Frequency	Weighted Criticality Score
Demonstrate knowledge of established and evolving biomedical, clinical, epidemiological, and social-behavioral sciences, as well as the application of this knowledge to patient care.	4.3	4.3	13.0
Apply understanding of prosthetic technology and how this informs surgical decisions.	4.0	4.0	12.0
Have ability to identify and treat bursitis.	2.8	3.3	8.8
Low Agreement			
Have ability to appraise and assimilate scientific evidence.[c]	4.0	4.7	12.7
Apply understanding of heterotopic ossification and subsequent surgical management.[c]	3.7	4.3	11.7
Demonstrate familiarity with signs and symptoms associated with failure of myodesis and loss of soft tissue padding, and when surgical revision is indicated.[c]	3.7	4.3	11.7
Apply understanding of skin problems at the skin-prosthesis interface and ability to provide surgical management (e.g., skin grafts) as necessary.[c]	3.7	4.3	11.7
Apply understanding of heterotopic ossification and subsequent surgical management.[c]	3.7	4.3	11.7
Understand nonoperative and less invasive modalities useful for treatment of residual limb and neuroma pain.[b]	3.7	4.0	11.3
Be aware of new prosthetic options for amputees.[b]	3.7	3.7	11.0
Apply understanding of the management of burn-related amputations and use of skin grafts.[c]	3.3	4.0	10.7
Competency: Ethical and Professional Behavior			
High Agreement			
Demonstrate commitment to carrying out professional responsibilities and an adherence to ethical principles.	5.0	5.0	15.0
Respect patient privacy and autonomy.	4.5	4.5	13.5

Table E.6—Continued

	Mean Importance	Mean Frequency	Weighted Criticality Score
Have ability to investigate and evaluate care of patients and to continuously improve patient care based on constant self-evaluation and lifelong learning.	4.3	4.5	13.0
Low Agreement			
Demonstrate awareness of and responsiveness to the larger context and system of health care.[c]	3.7	4.0	11.3

NOTES:
[b] Indicates items that were proposed in the first survey and therefore were rated only once (in the second survey).
[c] Reflects items that had <70 percent agreement in the first survey.

IMPORTANCE scale ranges from 1 (not important) to 5 (critically important); frequency scale ranges from 1 (never) to 5 (all the time). Responses listed in table reflect the results of the second survey. If the item reached the agreement threshold after the second survey, it is no longer classified as low agreement.

Table E.7
Physical Therapy Technical Expert Survey on Competencies for Amputation Rehabilitation

	Mean Importance	Mean Frequency	Weighted Criticality Score
Competency: Teamwork			
High Agreement			
Collaborate with members of the multidisciplinary rehabilitation team.	4.9	4.8	14.5
Establish and monitor a plan of care in consultation, cooperation, and collaboration with other involved health care team members to ensure that care is continuous and reliable.	4.9	4.5	14.3
Apply interpersonal and communication skills to interactions with other providers.	4.6	4.6	13.9
Provide leadership and supervision to PT assistants and direction for care.	4.3	3.8	12.3
Competency: Patient and Family Education			
High Agreement			
Educate the patient on how to don and doff a liner and a prosthesis.[b]	5.0	4.7	14.7
Teach the patient the componentry of the prosthetic and how to use and clean a prosthetic.	4.9	4.6	14.4
Teach patients rehabilitation exercises.	4.8	4.8	14.3
Educate patients, family, and caregivers using relevant and effective teaching methods to ensure optimal patient care outcomes.	4.8	4.5	14.0
Educate patient and family members about the goals and course of rehabilitation.	4.5	4.8	13.8
Educate the patient on the appropriate fit of the prosthesis.[b]	4.7	4.3	13.7
Educate the patient on appropriate shoes to wear with prosthesis.[b]	4.0	4.3	12.3
Low Agreement			
Educate the patient on the management of sweat.[b]	4.7	4.3	13.7

Table E.7—Continued

	Mean Importance	Mean Frequency	Weighted Criticality Score
Educate the patient on maintenance of the prosthesis.[b]	4.7	3.7	13.0
Educate the patient on appropriate adaptive clothing.[b]	3.0	3.0	9.0
Competency: Military and Other Cultural Awareness			
High Agreement			
Demonstrate comfort touching a residual limb.	4.4	4.4	13.1
Understand the unique needs and preferences of a military patient population with regard to rehabilitation.	4.4	3.9	12.6
Low Agreement			
Apply the orthopaedic sports medicine model to return service members to optimal levels of physical function.[c]	3.3	3.0	9.7
Competency: Patient-Centered Care			
High Agreement			
Establish and monitor a plan of care in consultation, cooperation, and collaboration with the patient.	4.6	4.8	14.0
Creatively adapt and modify exercises to allow patient to succeed.	4.5	4.5	13.5
Develop rapport with patients and family members.	4.4	4.6	13.4
Be a problem solver to meet the specific needs of the patient.[c]	4.3	4.7	13.3
Plan for discharge in consultation with the patient and caregivers.	4.4	4.5	13.3
Demonstrate strong communication skills for interacting with the patient and family members.	4.4	4.5	13.3
Respond to patients' emotional states.	4.5	4.3	13.3

Table E.7—Continued

	Mean Importance	Mean Frequency	Weighted Criticality Score
Understand the end state level of function (e.g., exercise, recreation, hobbies) that the individual aims to achieve for personal fulfillment.†	4.3	4.7	13.3
Provide support to patients as they navigate frustrations.	4.5	4.1	13.1
Manage patient expectations.	4.4	4.3	13.0
Collaborate with patient to update rehabilitation goals throughout the course of rehabilitation.	4.5	4.0	13.0
Be compassionate and personable.	4.1	4.6	12.9
Build a therapeutic relationship with patients.	4.1	4.6	12.9
Encourage the patient to create motivation and buy-in for therapy.	4.3	4.3	12.8
Be a patient advocate.	4.3	4.1	12.6
Low Agreement			
Understand and implement appropriate adaptations to exercises.[b]	4.3	4.3	13.0
Be adaptable and able to modify or apply protocols as needed to suit the needs of an individual patient.[b]	3.7	4.3	11.7
Locate local resources.[b]	3.7	4.0	11.3
Understand the functional demands of the individual's career field.[b]	3.7	4.0	11.3
Competency: Evidence-Based Practice			
High Agreement			
Understand how a prosthesis is designed to ascend/descend stairs/ramps in order to properly educate the patient.[b]	5.0	4.7	14.7
Implement rehabilitation exercises to promote functional activities, flexibility, strengthening, cardiovascular endurance, balance, ambulation, and other skills needed to return to work/recreation.	4.8	4.9	14.4

Table E.7—Continued

	Mean Importance	Mean Frequency	Weighted Criticality Score
Apply knowledge of clinical skills (e.g., gait training skills, observational gait analysis).	4.6	4.8	14.0
Understand how each prosthesis works.[t]	4.7	4.7	14.0
Consistently integrate the best evidence for practice from all sources of information and utilize clinical judgment to determine the best care for a patient.	4.6	4.6	13.9
Implement clinical evaluation techniques.	4.6	4.6	13.9
Demonstrate lifelong learning to identify, acquire, and apply knowledge, skills, and abilities required for current PT practice.	4.5	4.5	13.5
Deliver, evaluate, and adjust the PT intervention.	4.4	4.6	13.4
Choose the most appropriate outcomes measure for the patient.[b]	4.3	4.7	13.3
Apply understanding of available functional outcomes measures.[b]	4.0	4.7	12.7
Low Agreement			
Demonstrate skills to fit a prosthesis.[c]	4.7	4.0	13.3
Understand and implement appropriate therapeutic interventions.[b]	4.3	4.7	13.3
Understand which muscles to lengthen and which to strengthen to provide the most symmetrical gait patterns.[b]	4.3	4.7	13.3
Develop and implement a wear schedule for the prosthesis.[b]	4.7	3.7	13.0
Understand and implement proper therapeutic interventions to decrease back pain and prolong prosthetic wear.[b]	4.0	4.3	12.3
Understand the ways that the gait, deviations, and musculature of a patient with limb loss differ from other orthopaedic issues.[b]	3.7	4.3	11.7
Demonstrate manual therapy skills.[c]	3.7	3.3	10.7

Table E.7—Continued

	Mean Importance	Mean Frequency	Weighted Criticality Score
Demonstrate skills for inpatient rehabilitation.[c]	3.7	2.3	9.7
Competency: Ethical and Professional Behavior			
High Agreement			
Practice in a safe manner that minimizes risk to patients, self, and others.	4.9	5.0	14.8
Conduct critical self-assessment in order to practice to the fullest extent of knowledge, skills, and abilities and take responsibility to make accommodations as necessary.	4.5	4.4	13.4
Manage personal stress and personal responses and reactions to patient presenting concerns and injuries.	4.3	4.1	12.6

NOTES:
[b] Indicates items that were proposed in the first survey and therefore were rated only once (in the second survey).
[c] Reflects items that had <70 percent agreement in the first survey.

IMPORTANCE scale ranges from 1 (not important) to 5 (critically important); frequency scale ranges from 1 (never) to 5 (all the time). Responses listed in table reflect the results of the second survey. If the item reached the agreement threshold after the second survey, it is no longer classified as low agreement.

Table E.8
Physical Medicine and Rehabilitation Technical Expert Survey on Competencies for Amputation Rehabilitation

	Mean Importance	Mean Frequency	Weighted Criticality Score
Competency: Teamwork			
High Agreement			
Use interpersonal and communication skills that result in the effective exchange of information and collaboration with health professionals.	4.7	4.8	14.2
Effectively call on other resources in the system to provide optimal health care.	4.7	4.5	13.8
Lead the interdisciplinary team.	4.7	4.5	13.8
Low Agreement			
Communicate effectively with the interdisciplinary team to understand patient goals.[c]	4.2	4.5	12.8
Competency: Patient and Family Education			
High Agreement			
Explain common aftereffects of amputation to patients, including heterotopic ossification and phantom limb pain.[b]	5.0	5.0	15.0
Have ability to work with patients, providers, and family members on goal-setting and expectation management.	4.8	5.0	14.7
Communicate with family members, understand their role in patient's rehabilitation, and engage them in services as needed.	4.5	4.3	13.3
Competency: Military and Other Cultural Awareness			
High Agreement			
Demonstrate sensitivity and responsiveness to a diverse patient population, including but not limited to diversity in gender, age, culture, race, religion, disabilities, economic background, and sexual orientation.	4.3	4.5	13.2

Table E.8—Continued

	Mean Importance	Mean Frequency	Weighted Criticality Score
Low Agreement			
Demonstrate competence in the evaluation and treatment of patients of diverse backgrounds.[c]	4.2	4.3	12.7
Competency: Patient-Centered Care			
High Agreement			
Provide patient care that is compassionate, appropriate, and effective for the treatment of health problems and the promotion of health.	4.8	5.0	14.7
Demonstrate compassion, integrity, and respect for others.	4.8	5.0	14.7
Critically assess patient needs, wants, and progress versus challenges.	4.8	5.0	14.6
Develop a patient-centered care plan.	4.7	5.0	14.3
Demonstrate interpersonal and communication skills that result in the effective exchange of information and collaboration with patients and their families.	4.7	4.8	14.2
Be able to adapt to and be flexible regarding the clinical situation and individual patient needs.	4.5	4.8	13.8
Competency: Evidence-Based Practice			
High Agreement			
Evaluate nerve deficiencies that may affect the use of the amputated limb.[b]	5.0	5.0	15.0
Diagnose and treat pain conditions.[b]	5.0	5.0	15.0
Care for patients with musculoskeletal disorders in inpatient and outpatient settings.	4.8	4.7	14.3
Assess impairment and provide prescriptions for assistive technology.	4.7	4.8	14.2
Demonstrate understanding and knowledge of available prosthetic devices.[b]	4.7	4.7	14.0

Table E.8—Continued

	Mean Importance	Mean Frequency	Weighted Criticality Score
Apply knowledge of prosthetic components and different indications for use.[b]	4.3	4.7	13.3
Demonstrate knowledge of behavioral and mental health.	4.3	4.3	13.0
Low Agreement			
Apply knowledge of wound care and dermatological issues related to amputation.[b]	4.7	4.3	13.7
Visually evaluate gait to make appropriate recommendations for the prosthetic or PT regimen.[b]	4.3	4.3	13.0
Apply knowledge of gait biomechanics in amputee care.[b]	4.3	4.3	13.0
Demonstrate knowledge of the principles of pharmacology and the complications associated with medications.[c]	4.3	4.5	13.2
Detect symptoms and behavioral changes associated with mild TBI.[b]	4.0	4.3	12.3
Diagnose and treat neuromusculoskeletal, neurobehavioral, and other system disorders using reliable, valid diagnostic techniques.[c]	4.2	4.0	12.3
Assess gait analysis studies.[b]	3.7	4.3	11.7
Perform all medical and diagnostic procedures considered essential for the area of practice.[c]	3.7	4.0	11.3
Demonstrate knowledge of established and evolving biomedical, clinical, epidemiological, and social-behavioral sciences, as well as the application of this knowledge to patient care.[c]	3.7	4.0	11.3
Appraise scientific evidence and integrate it into practice.[c]	3.3	4.0	10.7
Competency: Ethical and Professional Behavior			
High Agreement			
Demonstrate a commitment to carrying out professional responsibilities and an adherence to ethical principles.	5.0	5.0	15.0

Table E.8—Continued

	Mean Importance	Mean Frequency	Weighted Criticality Score
Investigate, evaluate, and continuously improve patient care based on constant self-evaluation and lifelong learning.	4.3	4.5	13.2
Be aware of and responsive to the larger context and system of health care.[c]	4.0	4.5	12.5

NOTES:
[b] Indicates items that were proposed in the first survey and therefore were rated only once (in the second survey).
[c] Reflects items that had <70 percent agreement in the first survey.

IMPORTANCE scale ranges from 1 (not important) to 5 (critically important); frequency scale ranges from 1 (never) to 5 (all the time). Responses listed in table reflect the results of the second survey. If the item reached the agreement threshold after the second survey, it is no longer classified as low agreement.

Table E.9
Prosthetics and Orthotics Technical Expert Survey on Competencies for Amputation Rehabilitation

	Mean Importance	Mean Frequency	Weighted Criticality Score
Competency: Teamwork			
High Agreement			
Comprehend and demonstrate knowledge of the collaborative role of the prosthetist/orthotist as a member of the interdisciplinary rehabilitation team in providing patient-centered care.	4.8	4.2	13.8
Collaborate with other team members to develop medical and rehabilitation care plans.	4.6	3.8	13.0
Demonstrate understanding of the skills and knowledge of other providers' disciplines to facilitate effective collaboration.[c]	3.8	3.8	11.3
Low Agreement			
Communicate and work with interdisciplinary team members, including providing education and guidance/recommendations.[c]	3.7	3.7	11.0
Competency: Patient and Family Education			
High Agreement			
Provide education to patients on how to use a prosthetic device, including donning and doffing, different application techniques, and battery insertion, charging, and care.	4.8	4.6	14.2
Provide education to patients to enable informed decisionmaking.	4.4	4.0	12.8
Demonstrate the ability to impart knowledge when providing learning services for patients and their families, other health professionals and the public at large.[c]	4.3	4.0	12.5
Competency: Military and Other Cultural Awareness			
High Agreement			
Demonstrate an awareness of the humanity and dignity of all patients and related individuals within a diverse and multicultural society.	4.6	4.6	13.8

Table E.9—Continued

	Mean Importance	Mean Frequency	Weighted Criticality Score
Competency: Patient-Centered Care			
High Agreement			
Collaborate with patients to understand patients' needs, functional and personal goals, values, and preferences.	4.8	4.6	14.2
Provide ethical patient-centered care by applying nationally accepted professional responsibilities in clinical practice experiences.[c]	4.8	4.5	14.0
Demonstrate the ability to make clinical decisions designed to meet patient expectations, as well as achieve prescribed orthotic or prosthetic outcomes.	4.6	4.2	13.4
Communicate effectively with patients in order to balance patient ideas and goals with evidence-based interventions.	4.4	4.2	13.0
Be flexible regarding and adaptable to the clinical situation.	4.2	4.2	12.6
Competency: Evidence-Based Practice			
High Agreement			
Demonstrate proficiency in clinical and technical procedures that support practice.	4.8	4.2	13.8
Accommodate volumetric changes in the residual limb for individuals who have sustained blast wounds.	4.8	4.2	13.8
Demonstrate the technical ability to create prosthetic device, modify the device, and think creatively to determine which device works best for an individual patient.	4.6	4.4	13.6
Apply knowledge of available technology and programs for prosthetic devices.	4.4	4.0	12.8
Manage medical complications (e.g., swelling in the residual limb) to assist a patient's recovery.	4.4	4.0	12.8
Demonstrate the ability to integrate knowledge of the fundamental science of human function (physical, cognitive, social, psychological) with the practice framework of assessment, formulation, implementation, and follow-up of a comprehensive treatment plan.	4.0	4.2	12.2

Table E.9—Continued

	Mean Importance	Mean Frequency	Weighted Criticality Score
Demonstrate appropriate insight into clinical practice, clinical operations, and practice management within the social, cultural, and economic constructs of human function and disability.[c]	4.0	4.0	12
Low Agreement			
Apply knowledge of new and innovative prosthetic designs.[c]	4.2	3.8	12.2
Demonstrate the ability to participate as a critical consumer of research and to integrate research findings as evidence in clinical practice.[c]	3.8	2.8	10.3
Demonstrate the ability to participate in research activities through a working knowledge of the research process.[c]	3.3	2.5	9.0
Competency: Ethical and Professional Behavior			
High Agreement			
Adhere to safety procedures throughout the delivery of services.	5.0	4.6	14.6
Document pertinent information in a manner that promotes efficient direction for patient care, supports effective collegial communication, and meets the requirements of legal, business, and financial constraints.	4.6	4.6	13.8

NOTES:
[b] Indicates items that were proposed in the first survey and therefore were rated only once (in the second survey).
[c] Reflects items that had <70 percent agreement in the first survey.

IMPORTANCE scale ranges from 1 (not important) to 5 (critically important); frequency scale ranges from 1 (never) to 5 (all the time). Responses listed in table reflect the results of the second survey. If the item reached the agreement threshold after the second survey, it is no longer classified as low agreement.

Training and Education in Amputation Rehabilitation

In an effort to document the training and education that students in entry-level programs receive in amputation rehabilitation, we conducted informational interviews with universities and professors in the following educational disciplines:

- occupational therapy
- surgery
- physical therapy
- biomedical engineering
- social work
- clinical psychology
- psychiatry
- orthotist and prosthetist
- nutrition and dietitian
- physical medicine and rehabilitation.

We sent an invitation and two reminders to the top-rated 10–15 programs in each discipline ("Best Hospitals," undated). A total of 125 programs were invited to participate in a 15- to 30-minute interview to answer four questions:

1. What does your program teach students about amputation rehabilitation?
2. How do you teach them this? Didactic, hands-on, observation? [For MD programs, who was taught: Med students? Residents? Fellows?]
3. How much education or training do students receive in amputation rehabilitation? Frequency?
4. Can you provide us with an example syllabus that focuses on amputation rehabilitation?

Despite our reminders and comprehensive list of top programs, we encountered challenges in recruiting participants and received only 27 responses. We completed eight informational interviews, which included three in PM&R programs, one in a dietitian and nutritionist program, three in prosthetists and orthotists, and one in a PT program. A few programs replied that they did not currently include a course or teach on the subject of amputation rehabilitation. These programs were surgery (n = 1), biomedical engineering (n = 1), social work (n = 3), and nutritionist and dietitian (n = 1). One psychology program replied that they would not be participating in an interview, but they did teach a course on rehabilitation psychology and disability.

The informational interviews revealed an array of amputation rehabilitation courses. While we focused primarily on undergraduate courses to cast a wide net in terms of the programs we reached, we did include graduate and residency programs or components on amputation rehabilitation. The PM&R residency training program included a lecture series that covered the reasons for amputation, gait cycle, and prosthetics. Another PM&R program involved a multidisciplinary team that provided predoctoral internships and externships in clinical psychology. The internship involved lecture, observation, and supervised training with patients. The dietitian and nutritionist program did not explicitly provide training in amputation rehabilitation, but it did include lectures on trauma care and nutrition for wound healing.

The prosthetist and orthotist program interviews were unique because most of their programs are essentially focused on amputation rehabilitation. A program on transtibial and transfemoral prosthetics prepared entry-level clinicians mostly through didactic courses. Another program located within the PM&R Department had a Military provider teach a course specifically for high-level activity individuals. All of the programs that were interviewed mentioned that they taught their students based on the National Commission on Orthotic and Prosthetic Education (NCOPE) accreditation guidelines for the profession.

The PT program had a dedicated course on the management of persons with orthotics and prosthetics. The course was divided into lower-extremity and upper-extremity prosthetics. The program also included a course on amputation rehabilitation, which was a mix of lecture and lab; the latter included practicing limb wrapping, case studies, and reviewing componentry.

References

22 Kill, "22 Kill: About," undated. As of August 22, 2018:
http://www.22kill.com/about/#/

Accreditation Council for Graduate Medical Education, "Common Program Requirements," 2015.
As of March 12, 2019:
https://www.acgme.org/What-We-Do/Accreditation/Common-Program-Requirements

The American Occupational Therapy Association, "Standards of Practice," 2013. As of March 14,
2019:
https://www.pacificu.edu/sites/default/files/documents/Standards%20of%20Practice-2015.pdf

Association of American Medical Colleges, "New Research Shows Increasing Physician Shortages in
Both Primary and Specialty Care," April 11, 2018. As of July 12, 2018:
https://news.aamc.org/press-releases/article/workforce_report_shortage_04112018/

Association of Rehabilitation Nurses, "Become a Certified Rehabilitation Registered Nurse
(CRRN)," undated. As of August 22, 2018:
https://rehabnurse.org/crrn-certification/crrn-certification

Beebe, Gilbert W., and Michael E. DeBakey, *Battle Casualties: Incidence, Mortality, and Logistics
Considerations*, Springfield, Ill.: Thomas, 1952.

Bell, Elizabeth M., Alison L. Pruziner, et al., "Performance of Conventional and X2® Prosthetic
Knees During Slope Descent," *Clinical Biomechanics*, Vol. 33, 2016, pp. 26–31.

Berke, Gary M., John Fergason, et al., "Comparison of Satisfaction with Current Prosthetic Care in
Veterans and Servicemembers from Vietnam and OIF/OEF Conflicts with Major Traumatic Limb
Loss," *Journal of Rehabilitation Research & Development*, Vol. 47, No. 4, 2010, pp. 361–371.

"Best Hospitals for Rehabilitation," *U.S. News and World Report*, undated. As of August 24, 2018:
https://health.usnews.com/best-hospitals/rankings/rehabilitation

Birchall Blackburn Law, "Brain Injury Charity Pioneers Virtual Reality Rehabilitation for People
Living with Dementia," undated. As of March 22, 2019:
https://www.birchallblackburn.co.uk/brain-injury-charity-pioneers-virtual-reality-rehabilitation-for
-people-living-with-dementia/

Blough, David K., Sharon Hubbard, et al., "Prosthetic Cost Projections for Servicemembers with
Major Limb Loss from Vietnam and OIF/OEF," *Journal of Rehabilitation Research & Development*,
Vol. 47, No. 4, 2010, pp. 387–402.

Bush, George W., remarks to medical personnel at Walter Reed Army Medical Center, Office of the
Press Secretary release, Walter Reed Army Medical Center, Washington, D.C., December 18, 2003.

Carino, Michael, *Army Casualty: Summary Statistics*, Falls Church, Va.: Office of the Surgeon General of the Army, Program Analysis & Evaluation Office, February 12, 2016a.

Carino, Michael, *Army Casualty: Summary Statistics Overview—Update*, Falls Church, Va.: Office of the Surgeon General of the Army, Program Analysis & Evaluation Office, March 2016b.

Case Management Society of America, Standards of Practice for Case Management, 2016. As of February 23, 2019:
https://www.miccsi.org/wp-content/uploads/2017/03/CMSA-Standards-2016.pdf

Cheek, Gary, *Army Wounded Warrior Program (AW2): 5th Anniversary Report 2004–2009*, Alexandria, Va.: U.S. Army Wounded Warrior Program (AW2), 2009.

Cheesborough, Jennifer E., Lauren H. Smith, et al., "Targeted Muscle Reinnervation and Advanced Prosthetic Arms," *Seminars in Plastic Surgery*, Vol. 29, No. 1, 2015, pp. 62–72.

Cherry, Bobby, "Amputee Center Cost," Navy Medical Center San Diego, 2005.

Clay-Williams, R., and J. Braithwaite, "Determination of Health-Care Teamwork Training Competencies: A Delphi Study," *International Journal for Quality in Health Care*, Vol. 21, No. 6, 2009, pp. 433–440.

Coleman, C. A., S. Hudson, and L. L. Maine, "Health Literacy Practices and Educational Competencies for Health Professionals: A Consensus Study," *Journal of Health Communication*, Vol. 18, Supplement 1, 2013, pp. 82–102.

DARPA—*See* Defense Advanced Research Projects Agency.

Defense Advanced Research Projects Agency, "DARPA Provides Mobius Bionics LUKE Arms to Walter Reed: First Production Versions of Groundbreaking Upper-Limb Prostheses Becoming Available to Military Amputees," Washington, D.C., 2016.

Defense Casualty Analysis System, *Casualty Summary by Casualty Category*, Defense Manpower Data Center, Defense Casualty Analysis System, February 2, 2017.

Defense Health Board, *Sustainment and Advancement of Amputee Care*, Falls Church, Va., 2015.

Department of Veterans Affairs, Office of Rehabilitation Research and Development, "Survey for Prosthetic Use," undated. As of March 22, 2019:
https://www.rehab.research.va.gov/jour/10/474/pdf/prostheticssurvey.pdf

DHB—*See* Defense Health Board.

DOD—*See* U.S. Department of Defense.

Dougherty, Paul J., Lynne V. McFarland, et al., "Multiple Traumatic Limb Loss: A Comparison of Vietnam Veterans to OIF/ OEF Servicemembers," *Journal of Rehabilitation Research & Development*, Vol. 47, No. 4, 2010, pp. 333–348.

Doukas, William C., "Information Paper: Amputee Care Center—Summary of Current Plan for Battle Casualty Research at WRAMC," 2003.

Drauden, G. M., "Task Inventory Analysis in Industry and the Public Sector," in S. Gael, ed., *The Job Analysis Handbook for Business, Industry, and Government*, Vol. 2, New York: John Wiley & Sons, 1988, pp. 1051–1071.

Driever, M. J. "Are Evidenced-Based Practice and Best Practice the Same?" *Western Journal of Nursing Research*, Vol. 24, No. 5, 2002, pp. 591–597.

EACE—*See* Extremity Trauma and Amputation Center of Excellence.

Epstein, Richard A., Allen W. Heinemann, and Lynne V. McFarland, "Quality of Life for Veterans and Servicemembers with Major Traumatic Limb Loss from Vietnam and OIF/OEF Conflicts," *Journal of Rehabilitation Research & Development*, Vol. 47, No. 4, 2010, pp. 373–386.

Extremity Trauma and Amputation Center of Excellence, "EACE Overview," Defense Health Agency, Falls Church, Va., undated. As of April 17, 2017:
https://health.mil/EACE

Federation of State Boards of Physical Therapy, "Standards of Competence," October 19, 2006. As of February 23, 2019:
https://www.fsbpt.org/Portals/0/Content%20Manager/PDFs/free-resources/StandardsOf
Competence2006_10.pdf

Figg, Laurann, and Jane Farrell-Beck, "Amputation in the Civil War: Physical and Social Dimensions," *Journal of the History of Medicine and Allied Sciences*, Vol. 48, 1993, pp. 454–475.

Fischer, Hannah, *A Guide to U.S. Military Casualty Statistics: Operation Freedom's Sentinel, Operation Inherent Resolve, Operation New Dawn, Operation Iraqi Freedom, and Operation Enduring Freedom*, Washington, D.C.: Congressional Research Service, 2015.

Gailey, Robert, Lynne V. McFarland, et al., "Unilateral Lower-Limb Loss: Prosthetic Device Use and Functional Outcomes in Servicemembers from Vietnam War and OIF/OEF Conflicts," *Journal of Rehabilitation Research & Development*, Vol. 47, No. 4, 2010, pp. 317–332.

Geertzen, Jan H. B., G. M. Rommers, and Rienk Dekker, "An ICF-Based Education Programme in Amputation Rehabilitation for Medical Residents in the Netherlands," *Prosthetics and Orthotics International*, Vol. 35, No. 3, 2011, pp. 318–322.

Government of South Australia, "Lifetime Support: Guidelines for Treatment, Care and Support for Amputees Within the LSS Living in the Community," undated. As of February 23, 2019:
http://lifetimesupport.sa.gov.au/wp-content/uploads/Amputee-Framework-Guidelines.pdf

Hafner, Brian J., Laura L. Willingham, et al., "Evaluation of Function, Performance, and Preference as Transfemoral Amputees Transition from Mechanical to Microprocessor Control of the Prosthetic Knee," *Archives of Physical Medical Rehabilitation*, Vol. 88, 2007, pp. 207–217.

Hampton, Oscar P., Jr, *Orthopedic Surgery in the Mediterranean Theater of Operations*, Washington, D.C.: Office of the Surgeon General, Department of the Army, 1957.

Health.mil, "Competency Assessment File," undated. As of March 15, 2019:
https://health.mil/Military-Health-Topics/Health-Readiness/Immunization-Healthcare/Education
-and-Training/Guidelines/Competency-Assessment-File

Highsmith, M. Jason, and Jason T. Kahle, "Getting the Most out of Physical Therapy," *InMotion*, Vol. 18, No. 6, 2008, pp. 30–34.

Hooper, Rebecca S. "Information Paper: Center for the Intrepid at Brooke Army Medical Center," Office of the Surgeon General of the Army, 2007.

Hudak, Ronald P., Christine Morrison, et al., "The U.S. Army Wounded Warrior Program (AW2): A Case Study in Designing a Nonmedical Case Management Program for Severely Wounded, Injured, and Ill Service Members and Their Families," *Military Medicine*, Vol. 174, No. 6, 2009, pp. 566–571.

Hurley, Richard K., Jessica C. Rivera, et al., "Identifying Obstacles to Return to Duty in Severely Injured Combat-Related Servicemembers with Amputation," *Journal of Rehabilitation Research & Development*, Vol. 52, No. 1, 2015, pp. 53–61.

The Institute for Rehabilitation and Research Memorial Hermann, "TIRR Memorial Hermann 2015 Facts," undated-a. As of August 22, 2018:
http://tirr.memorialhermann.org/programs-specialties/outcomes/

The Institute for Rehabilitation and Research Memorial Hermann, "Traumatic Brain Injury Model System," undated-b. As of August 22, 2018:
http://tirr.memorialhermann.org/research/national-database/

Institute of Medicine (U.S.) Committee on the Health Professions Education Summit, A. C. Greiner and E. Knebel, eds., *Health Professions Education: A Bridge to Quality*, Washington, D.C., National Academies Press, 2003. As of March 14, 2019:
https://www.ncbi.nlm.nih.gov/books/NBK221528/pdf/Bookshelf_NBK221528.pdf

Isaacson, Brad M., Thomas M. Swanson, and Paul F. Pasquina, "The Use of a Computer-Assisted Rehabilitation Environment (CAREN) for Enhancing Wounded Warrior Rehabilitation Regimens," *Journal of Spinal Cord Medicine*, Vol. 36, No. 4, 2013, pp. 296–299.

Janke, K. K., K. A. Kelley, B. V. Sweet, and S. E. Kuba, "A Modified Delphi Process to Define Competencies for Assessment Leads Supporting a Doctor of Pharmacy Program," *American Journal of Pharmaceutical Education*, Vol. 80, No. 10, 2016, p. 167. As of March 21, 2019:
https://experts.umn.edu/en/publications/a-modified-delphi-process-to-define-competencies-for-assessment-l

Johns Hopkins Applied Physics Laboratory, "Prosthetics: The Program," undated. As of February 23, 2019:
https://www.jhuapl.edu/prosthetics/program/default.asp

Kak, Neeraj, Bart Burkhalter, and Merri-Ann Cooper, *Measuring the Competence of Healthcare Providers*, Bethesda, Md.: Published for the U.S. Agency for International Development (USAID) by the Quality Assurance (QA) Project, Operations Research Issue Paper 2(1), 2001.

Kapp, Susan, and Joseph A. Miller, "Lower Limb Prosthetics," in Martha K. Lenhart, Col. Paul F. Pasquina M.D., and Rory A. Cooper, ed., *Care of the Combat Amputee*, Walter Reed Army Medical Center, Washington, D.C.: Borden Institute, 2009.

Kishbaugh, David, Timothy R. Dillingham, Robin S. Howard, Melissa W. Sinnott, and Praxedes V. Belandres, "Amputee Soldiers and Their Return to Active Duty," *Military Medicine*, Vol. 160, 1995, pp. 82–84.

Koebler, Jason, "New Prosthetics Keep Amputee Soldiers on Active Duty: Technology Advances—and Strong Willpower—Have Allowed Some Injured Soldiers to Return to Battle," *U.S. News and World Report*, May 25, 2012. As of February 23, 2019:
https://www.usnews.com/news/articles/2012/05/25/new-prosthetics-keep-amputee-soldiers-on-active-duty

Krueger, Chad A., Joseph C. Wenke, and James R. Ficke, "Ten Years at War: Comprehensive Analysis of Amputation Trends," *Journal of Trauma and Acute Care Surgery*, Vol. 73, No. 6, Supplement 5, 2012, pp. S438–S444.

Lenhart, Martha K., Col. Paul F. Pasquina M.D., and Rory A. Cooper, ed., *Care of the Combat Amputee*, Washington, D.C.: Walter Reed Army Medical Center, Borden Institute, 2009.

Levine, Adele, "The Day the Boston Bombings Sent a Shockwave Through Walter Reed," *Washington Post*, April 24, 2014.

Marrelli, A. F., J. Tondora, and M. A. Hoge, "Strategies for Developing Competency Models," *Administration and Policy in Mental Health*, Vol. 32, Nos. 5–6, 2005, pp. 533–561.

McFarland, Lynne V., Sandra L. Hubbard Winkler, et al., "Unilateral Upper-Limb Loss: Satisfaction and Prosthetic-Device Use in Veterans and Servicemembers from Vietnam and OIF/OEF Conflicts," *Journal of Rehabilitation Research & Development*, Vol. 47, No. 4, 2010, pp. 299–316.

McHale, Kathleen A., "Care of War Amputees," Memorandum for the Surgeon General, Washington, D.C., October 11, 2001a.

McHale, Kathleen A., *Memorandum: Care of War Amputees*, Washington, D.C.: Army Office of the Surgeon General, 2001b.

Messinger, Seth D. "Incorporating the Prosthetic: Traumatic Limb-Loss, Rehabilitation and Refigured Military Bodies," *Disability and Rehabilitation*, Vol. 25, No. 31, 2019, pp. 2130–2134.

Miles, Donna, *Disabled Soldier Support System Helping Wounded Troops*, American Forces Press Service, Department of Defense, 2004.

The Military Health System, "Competency Assessment File," Defense Health Agency, Falls Church, Va., undated. As of March 15, 2019:
https://health.mil/Military-Health-Topics/Health-Readiness/Immunization-Healthcare/Education-and-Training/Guidelines/Competency-Assessment-File

The Military Health System, *The Military Health System Strategic Plan: Achieving a Better, Stronger, and More Relevant Military Health System*, 2014. As of March 15, 2019:
http://medxellence.pesgce.com/PreReads/2_Mon_PWSession_7_2015_2020_MHS_Strategic_Plan_Final_20141204_VF_3_2.pdf

Miller, Joseph A., *Executive Summary: Advanced Prosthetic Technologies*, Bethesda, Md.: Walter Reed Medical Center–Amputee Care Center, December 6, 2004.

Murray, Elizabeth, Shaun Treweek, et al., "Normalisation Process Theory: A Framework for Developing, Evaluating and Implementing Complex Interventions," *BioMed Central Medicine*, Vol. 8, No. 63, 2010, pp. 1–11.

National Academies of Sciences, Engineering, and Medicine, *A National Trauma Care System: Integrating Military and Civilian Trauma Systems to Achieve Zero Preventable Deaths After Injury*, Washington, D.C.: The National Academies Press, 2016. As of February 23, 2019:
doi: 10.17226/23511

National Commission on Orthotic and Prosthetic Education, *Core Curriculum for Orthotists and Prosthetists*, 2010. As of February 23, 2019:
http://www.ncope.org/view/?file=core_guide_for_OP

Navy Medical Center San Diego," Comprehensive Combat and Complex Casualty Care," undated. As of April 11, 2017:
http://www.med.navy.mil/sites/nmcsd/Pages/Care/C5.aspx

NMCSD—*See* Navy Medical Center San Diego.

Nottingham, Elizabeth, Jennifer Aldridge, et al., "Temporospatial Outcomes During Slope Ascent and Descent While Using a Novel Microprocessor Knee," paper presented at the 17th Annual Meeting of the Gait and Clinical Movement Analysis, May 2012, Grand Rapids, Mich.

Otis, George A., and D. L. Huntington, *The Medical and Surgical History of the War of the Rebellion, Part III*, Vol. II: *Surgical History*, Washington, D.C.: Government Printing Office, 1883. As of February 23, 2019:
http://ia311535.us.archive.org/1/items/medicalsurgical32barnrich/medicalsurgical32barnrich.pdf

Pasquina, Paul F., "DOD Paradigm Shift in Care of Servicemembers with Major Limb Loss," *Journal of Rehabilitation Research & Development Loss*, Vol. 47, No. 4, 2010, pp. xi–xiv.

Pasquina, Paul F., Charles R. Scoville, Brian Belnap, and Rory A. Cooper, "Introduction: Developing a System of Care for the Combat Amputee in Care of the Combat Amputee," in Martha K. Lenhart, Col. Paul F. Pasquina M.D., and Rory A. Cooper, ed., *Care of the Combat Amputee*, Washington, D.C.: Walter Reed Army Medical Center, Borden Institute, 2009.

Polly, David W., *The U.S. Army Amputee Care Program*, Bethesda, Md.: Walter Reed Medical Center–Amputee Care Center, 2003.

Poston, Walker S. C., Christopher K. Haddock, et al., "What Do Veterans Service Organizations' Web Sites Say About Tobacco Control?" *American Journal of Health Promotion*, Vol. 28, No. 2, 2013, pp. 88–96.

Public Law 110-417, Duncan Hunter National Defense Authorization Act for Fiscal Year 2009, October 14, 2008.

Public Law 114-328, National Defense Authorization Act for Fiscal Year 2017, December 23, 2016.

Pynes, J. E., *Human Resources Management for Public and Nonprofit Organizations: A Strategic Approach*, San Francisco, Calif.: John Wiley and Sons, 2009.

Reiber, Gayle E., Lynne V. McFarland, et al., "Servicemembers and Veterans with Major Traumatic Limb Loss from Vietnam War and OIF/OEF Conflicts: Survey Methods, Participants, and Summary Findings," *Journal of Rehabilitation Research & Development*, Vol. 47, No. 4, 2010, pp. 275–297.

Reister, Frank A., *Battle Casualties and Medical Statistics: U.S. Army Experience in the Korea War*, Washington, D.C.: Office of the Surgeon General, Department of the Army, 1973.

Reister, Frank A., *Medical Statistics in World War II*, Washington, D.C.: Office of the Surgeon General, Department of the Army, 1975.

Royal College of Physicians and Surgeons of Canada, "Competence by Design," undated. As of April 4, 2019:
http://www.royalcollege.ca/rcsite/cbd/competence-by-design-cbd-e

Sanchez, Justin, *Revolutionizing Prosthetics*, Washington, D.C.: Defense Advanced Research Projects Agency, 2017.

Sanders, Roy, and David Helfet, "The Choice Between Limb Salvage and Amputation: Trauma," in D. G. Smith, J. W. Michael, and J. H. Bowker, eds., *Atlas of Limb Prosthetics: Surgical, Prosthetic, and Rehabilitation Principles*, Rosemont, Ill.: American Academy of Orthopedic Surgeons, 2004.

Sasahara, T., Y. Kizawa, T. Morita, et al., "Development of a Standard for Hospital-Based Palliative Care Consultation Teams Using a Modified Delphi Method," *Journal of Pain and Symptom Management*, Vol. 38, No. 4, 2009, pp. 496–504.

Scales, Robert H. Jr., *Certain Victory: United States Army in the Gulf War*, Office of the Chief of Staff, United States Army, Washington, D.C., 1993.

Scoville, Charles, *Draft EXSUM: Recommendations for Care of War Amputees*, Washington, D.C.: Office of the Surgeon General of the Army, 2001a.

Scoville, Charles, *Information Paper: Amputee Care—Summary of Current Plan for the Care of Amputee Patients*, Washington, D.C.: Office of the Surgeon General of the Army, 2001b.

Scoville, Charles, "Care of Active Duty Persons with Lower Limb Amputations at a MEDCEN," Bethesda, Md.: Walter Reed Medical Center–Amputee Patient Care Center, 2002a.

Scoville, Charles, *Guidelines for Managements of War Amputees: A Uniform Approach to Treatment of Patients Requiring Amputation of an Extremity Following War Trauma*, Bethesda, Md.: Walter Reed Medical Center–Amputee Patient Care Center, 2002b.

Scoville, Charles, *Information Paper: Amputee Care Center—Updated Information to the Amputee Patient Care Board of Directors*, Washington, D.C.: Walter Reed Medical Center–Amputee Patient Care Center, 2003a.

Scoville, Charles, *Information Paper: Amputee Patient Registry and Follow Up Programs*, Bethesda, Md.: Walter Reed Medical Center–Amputee Care Center, 2003b.

Scoville, Charles, "Information Paper: Army and VA Collaboration on Amputee Care," Washington, D.C.: Walter Reed Medical Center–Amputee Care Center, 2003c.

Scoville, Charles, "Information Paper: U.S. Army Amputee Patient Care Program Update," Washington, D.C.: Walter Reed Medical Center–Amputee Patient Care Center, 2003d.

Scoville, Charles, "Information Paper: The Team Approach to Amputee Rehabilitation," Bethesda, Md.: Walter Reed Medical Center–Amputee Care Center, October 29, 2003e.

Scoville, Charles, *Information Paper: Walter Reed Amputee Center Infrastructure Improvement Plan*, Bethesda, Md.: Walter Reed Medical Center–Amputee Patient Care Center, 2003f.

Scoville, Charles, *Wounding Patterns Resulting from Military Conflict*, Bethesda, Md.: Walter Reed Medical Center–Amputee Patient Care Center, 2003g.

Scoville, Charles, "Information Paper: Military Amputee Patient Care Program—Respond to a Congressional Request for Information Regarding the Military Amputee Patient Care Program (MAPCP) Headquartered at Walter Reed Army Medical Center," Bethesda, Md.: Walter Reed Medical Center, 2004a.

Scoville, Charles, "Information Paper: Military Amputee Patient Care Program—Update on Amputee Patient Care," Bethesda, Md.: Walter Reed Medical Center–Amputee Patient Care Center, 2004b.

Scoville, Charles, *Infrastructure Improvement for the U.S. Army Amputee Patient Care Program: Report to Congress*, Bethesda, Md.: Walter Reed Medical Center–Amputee Patient Care Center, 2004b.

Scoville, Charles, *Prosthetic Costs*, Bethesda, Md.: Walter Reed Medical Center–Amputee Patient Care Center, 2004d.

Scoville, Charles, *VHA/ORD New and Ongoing Initiatives for Improving Health and Healthcare of Veterans with Limb Loss*, Bethesda, Md.: Walter Reed Medical Center–Amputee Patient Care Center, 2004e.

Scoville, Charles, *Executive Summary: Fisher Foundation*, Bethesda, Md.: Walter Reed Medical Center–Amputee Care Center, 2005a.

Scoville, Charles, *Executive Summary: Fisher Foundation II*, Bethesda, Md.: Walter Reed Medical Center–Amputee Care Center, 2005b.

Scoville, Charles, "Information Paper: Current Information on the Amputee Patient Care Program," Washington, D.C.: Walter Reed Medical Center–Amputee Care Center, 2005c.

Scoville, Charles, "Information Paper: Walter Reed Army Medical Center (WRAMC) Military Amputee Training Center (MATC) Project," Bethesda, Md.: Walter Reed Medical Center–Amputee Care Center, 2005d.

Scoville, Charles, *Amputee Patient Care*, Washington, D.C.: Office of the Surgeon General of the Army, 2006a.

Scoville, Charles, "Information Paper: Military Amputee Training Center (MATC) Project and BRAC," Bethesda, Md.: Walter Reed Medical Center–Amputee Care Center, 2006b.

Scoville, Charles, "Information Paper: Military Amputee Training Center (MATC) Project and BRAC II," Bethesda, Md.: Walter Reed Medical Center–Amputee Care Center, 2006c.

Scoville, Charles, *Armed Forces Amputee Patient Care Program: Briefing Presented at the Annual Meeting of the American College of Sports Medicine*, Washington, D.C.: Walter Reed Army Medical Center, 2007a.

Scoville, Charles, "Information Paper: Current Information on the Amputee Patient Care," Bethesda, Md.: Walter Reed Medical Center–Amputee Care Center, 2007b.

Scoville, Charles, "Information Paper: Military Advanced Training Center," Walter Reed Army Medical Center, Walter Reed Medical Center–Amputee Care Center, 2007c.

Shepherd Center, "About Shepherd Center," undated-a. As of August 22, 2018: https://www.shepherd.org/about/about-shepherd

Shepherd Center, "Beyond Therapy," undated-b. As of August 24, 2018: https://www.shepherd.org/patient-programs/beyond-therapy

Shepherd Center, "Brain Injury Care for U.S. Service Members," undated-c. As of August 22, 2018: https://www.shepherd.org/patient-programs/care-for-us-service-members

Shepherd Center, "Shepherd Center Sports," undated-d. As of August 22, 2018: https://www.shepherd.org/resources/sports

Shirley Ryan AbilityLab, "Adaptive Sports & Fitness Membership," undated-a. As of August 22, 2018: https://www.sralab.org/adaptive-sports-fitness-membership

Shirley Ryan AbilityLab, "LIFE Center," undated-b. As of August 22, 2018: https://www.sralab.org/lifecenter

Shirley Ryan AbilityLab, "Limb Loss + Impairment," undated-c. As of August 22, 2018: https://www.sralab.org/conditions/limb-loss-impairment

Shirley Ryan AbilityLab, "Peer Mentor Program at the Shirley Ryan Ability Lab," May 20, 2018. As of August 22, 2018: https://www.sralab.org/lifecenter/resources/PeerMentorProgram

Schippmann, J. S., R. A. Ash, M. Battista, L. Carr, L. D. Eyde, B. Hesketh, et al., "The Practice of Competency Modeling," *Personnel Psychology*, Vol. 53, 2000, pp. 703–740.

Stiers, W., M. Barisa, K. Stucky, C. Pawlowski, M. Van Tubbergen, A. P. Turner, M. Hibbard, and B. Caplan, "Guidelines for Competency Development and Measurement in Rehabilitation Psychology Postdoctoral Training," *Rehabilitation Psychology*, Vol. 60, 2015, pp. 111–122.

Sigford, Barbara J., "Paradigm Shift for VA Amputation Care," *Journal of Rehabilitation Research & Development*, Vol. 47, No. 4, 2010, pp. xv–xix.

Sinitski, Emily H., Edward D. Lemaire, and Natalie Baddour, "Evaluation of Motion Platform Embedded with Force Plate-Instrumented Treadmill," *Journal of Rehabilitation Research & Development*, Vol. 52, No. 2, 2015, pp. 221–234.

Sisson Mobility Restoration Center, "C-Leg." As of July 10, 2018: http://www.sissonmobility.com/c-leg/

Smith, Douglas G., and Gayle E. Reiber, "VA Paradigm Shift in Care of Veterans with Limb Loss," *Journal of Rehabilitation Research & Development*, Vol. 47, No. 4, 2010, pp. vii–x.

Society for Human Resource Management, "SHRM Competency Model," 2012. As of March 14, 2019:
https://www.shrm.org/LearningAndCareer/competency-model/Documents/Full%20Competency%20Model%2011%202_10%201%202014.pdf

Spaulding Rehabilitation Network, "Amputee Rehabilitation," undated-a. As of August 22, 2018: http://spauldingrehab.org/conditions-and-treatments/amputee-rehabilitation

Spaulding Rehabilitation Network, "Spaulding Rehabilitation Hospital Boston," undated-b. As of August 22, 2018:
http://spauldingrehab.org/locations/spaulding-rehabilitation-hospital/about

SRAL—*See* Shirley Ryan AbilityLab.

SRN—*See* Spaulding Rehabilitation Network.

St.-Jean, Carole, and Natalie Fish, "Osseointegration: Examining the Pros and Cons," *InMotion*, Vol. 21, No. 5, 2011, pp. 46–47.

Staff of Soldiers Magazine, "Disabled Soldier Support System," U.S. Army, May 1, 2005.

Stinner, Daniel J., Travis C. Burns, et al., "Return to Duty Rate of Amputee Soldiers in the Current Conflicts in Afghanistan and Iraq," *The Journal of Trauma*, Vol. 68, No. 6, 2010, pp. 1476–1479.

Strive Center, homepage, undated. As of March 15, 2019:
https://strive.ll.mit.edu/

Stutsky, Brenda J., Marilyn Singer, and Robert Renaud, "Determining the Weighting and Relative Importance of CanMEDS Roles and Competencies," *BMC Research Notes*, Vol. 5, 2012, pp. 1–7.

TIRR—*See* The Institute for Rehabilitation and Research Memorial Hermann.

University of Victoria, "Program Specific Competencies—Biomedical Engineering," undated. As of February 23, 2019:
https://www.uvic.ca/coopandcareer/assets/docs/student-docs/competencies/program-competencies/program_biomedical_engineering.pdf

U.S. Department of the Army, *Medical Services: Standards of Medical Fitness*, Army Regulation 40-501, August 29, 2003a. As of February 23, 2019:
http://www.au.af.mil/au/awc/awcgate/army/r40_501.pdf

U.S. Department of the Army, "Walter Reed Army Medical Center Charter of the Board of Directors, U.S. Army Amputee Patient Care Program," Walter Reed Army Medical Center, Washington, D.C., 2003b.

U.S. Department of the Army, *Medical Services: Standards of Medical Fitness*, Army Regulation 40-501, December 14, 2007. As of February 23, 2019:
https://deploymentpsych.org/system/files/member_resource/AR%2040-501.pdf

U.S. Department of Defense, "DoD Civilian Personnel Management System: Civilian Strategic Human Capital Planning (SHCP)," Department of Defense Instruction, Issue 1400.25, Vol. 250, June 7, 2016. As of February 23, 2019:
https://www.esd.whs.mil/Portals/54/Documents/DD/issuances/140025/140025_vol250.pdf

"Vietnam War Statistics," lzsally.com, 2015. As of August 24, 2018:
http://lzsally.com/archives/namfacts.html

Walter Reed National Military Medical Center, "Amputee Care," undated. As of April 12, 2017:
http://www.wrnmmc.capmed.mil/Health%20Services/Surgery/Orthopaedics%20and%20Rehabilitation/Amputee%20Care/SitePages/Home.aspx#CAREN

Werner, Kathryn M., Alison Linberg, and Erik J. Wolf, "Balance Recovery Kinematics After a Lateral Perturbation in Patients with Transfemoral Amputations," paper presented at the American Society of Biomechanics annual meeting, August 16, 2012, Gainesville, FL.

Wilson, J. R., "Prosthetics Meet Robotics," *Military & Aerospace Electronics*, October 8, 2013.

WRNMMC—*See* Walter Reed National Military Medical Center.

Yousuf, M. I., "Using Experts' Opinions Through Delphi Technique," *Practical Assessment, Research & Evaluation*, Vol. 12, No. 4, 2007, pp. 1–8.